SMALL GYM
BIG WORKOUTS

SMALL GYM
BIG WORKOUTS

MACK H. WEBB, JR.

PILINUT PRESS, INC

SMALL GYM
BIG WORKOUTS

Book and Cover Design by Celia Webb
Photographs by Mack H. Webb, Jr.

Pilinut Press, Inc.
www.pilinutpress.com

The Pilinut is the edible seed of the *Canarium ovatum* tree which is native to Southeast Asia. Tasting like sweet almonds, it is eaten for its health benefits including prevention of anemia and for nourishment of the brain and nervous system.

Library of Congress Control Number: 2014906502

Printed in Warrenton, Virginia

ISBN 978-0-9779576-9-9

TABLE OF CONTENTS

SMALL GYM
BIG WORKOUTS

1

INTRODUCTION

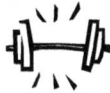

Small Gym Big Workouts assumes that you have already decided you want a home gym and it guides you through the process of obtaining equipment and setting up the gym.

Here are the topics which will be covered in this book:

- Why I feel there is a need for this book.
- Why workout at home?
- How much money is needed to outfit a home gym?
- How to get the money to outfit your home gym.
- Where in your home to set up your gym.
- Flooring options.
- Maximizing workout capability in small spaces.
- Mirror options.
- Storage space within your gym space.
- Basic equipment for your gym.
- Choosing a treadmill.
- Optional workout equipment.
- Nice-to-have accessories.
- Where to buy quality gym equipment.
- Where to get quality gym equipment for free.
- How to buy equipment.
- Equipment delivery versus hauling it yourself.
- Getting the equipment into your gym.
- Tools for setting up your equipment.
- Upkeep and maintenance procedures.
- Safety measures.
- Commercial and military gym etiquette.
- Exercise and technique examples.

Why I feel there is a need for this book

I am an Army brat and a veteran, who was bitten by the "barbell bug" in the late 1970's. Since then I have had the pleasure of working out in gyms in Brussels, Belgium; Canada; England; Germany; Korea; and 20 of the 50 states. Some of the gyms have been gems; some of them have been dumps.

Some of the problems I have encountered in gyms are:

- Not enough 45-pound weights to go around (I need as many as 22 for my super-heavy shrug exercise).
- They are so crammed with machines that it is difficult or impossible to find a place to do free-weight work.
- Lack of cleanliness.
- Terrible air quality (and someone is almost always hacking and sneezing with abandon).
- Weak barbells that sag as soon as you put more than 225 pounds on them.
- Some places don't allow weightlifting chalk. Outrageous!

Small Gym Big Workouts solves these problems and shows you how to design a home gym that meets your needs.

I've used just about every workout tool and apparatus on the market, and some home-made ones too. And what it all boils down to is you do not need a lot of big, cumbersome equipment in order to have an excellent workout.

3

Small Gym Big Workouts is geared around the workout equipment and accessories that I currently use in my home gym. Why this equipment? Because I know that you can get muscled, awesomely strong, control your bodyweight, and become cardiovascularly fit by using the equipment items listed here. I have put the equipment through years of rigorous workouts, and it has performed wonderfully. I will introduce you to each piece of equipment, explain why it is an important asset to the home gym, and describe the things you should look for or avoid when purchasing your own equipment. If you have your heart set on a piece of equipment other than what is covered in this book, not to worry. I will give you detailed information on how to choose any piece of equipment so that you will not be disappointed when you get it into your gym.

I am very thorough when covering each section. You will find that most, if not all, of your home gym questions are answered here.

I will cover exercises that are done using equipment that I already possess. The exercises I show will cover a full body workout.

With the amount of iron in my home gym, you may think it is off limits to my wife. Not so. My wife, a retired Army officer, uses the gym to stay healthy and svelte. This book is for men and women who want a home gym in which to manage their body weight, reshape their body, maintain their fitness, or go beyond their current fitness level.

Why workout at home?

There are many reasons why you would want to work out at home:

- Convenience. You won't have to worry about driving your vehicle to the gym in foul weather. Or driving at all for that matter, so you will save gas.
- Your gym will be open for you 24 hours a day, 7 days a week.
- You outfit your gym to your specifications, so you know that everything will be on hand to complete the workout you have in mind.
- There is no one present to talk your ear off. Your workouts will be more productive, and your workout time may decrease.
- You will not have to wait while someone else uses the piece of equipment you want to use.
- You are the boss and you set the gym rules.
- You can use weightlifting chalk.
- You no longer have to adhere to the 30 minute time limit for using cardio equipment.
- There is no one to tell you not to bang the weights (even so, don't bang the weights).
- You can grunt, strain, groan, and yell with abandon.

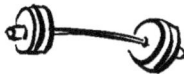

SMALL GYM BIG WORKOUTS

2

FINANCING YOUR GYM

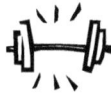

How much money is needed to outfit a home gym?

It cost $3,772.00 to set up my home gym. This dollar amount is for the basic equipment only.

- $159.00-Hampton 7-foot 1500# Olympic bar and two collars
- $40.00-2 Dumbbell handles with 2 sets of collars
- $2,299.00-Treadmill
- $39.99-Treadmill anti-static mat
- $299.99-ParaBody Multi-Angle Bench
- $349.00-Power Rack
- $317.08-Weight plates
- $89.95-Olympic weight plate tree
- $30.00-Shipping
- $147.99-Sales tax

Bear in mind the cost of certain pieces of equipment has gone up a little, but the price-hike is not excessive. Used equipment, if it is in excellent condition, should be considered as well. If possible, inspect the equipment before you purchase it.

The room that is now my gym first required that I install some electrical outlets (ground fault interrupt type), drywall sheets, and ceiling lights. I have not included the cost of these modifications. It would be hard to calculate costs since I did most of the work myself.

How to get the money to outfit a home gym

As boring as it may sound, you may want to work to raise the money for outfitting your gym. You will appreciate the gym more and it will give you a sense of pride. It is more likely that the equipment will receive loving care if you've had to toil to acquire it. There are, however, other ways to gather capital.

- Ask others for the money. If you have a birthday coming up, a holiday on which gifts are given, are graduating soon, or if your wedding is imminent request money instead of other gifts. You can also ask for the specific piece of gym equipment that you want or need. (In the case of weddings it's best to clear this with your prospective spouse first. No sense starting off on the wrong foot.)
- If you get an allowance, save some for buying gym equipment.
- You can always sell unwanted items that you have not used for years.
- You can get creative on e-bay. Ask for donations that will help you set up your gym. In exchange you can send your benefactors photo updates concerning your progress with and in your gym. Sound crazy? You may be surprised.
- Earn a bonus and use it to outfit your home gym.
- The military is currently giving thousands of dollars as signup bonuses. Okay, just a thought.

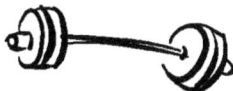

SMALL GYM BIG WORKOUTS

3

SELECTING GYM LOCATION

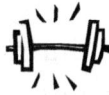

Where in the home to set up your gym

I set up my gym in the basement. I recommend you do the same if radon is not a problem. I chose the basement because I can lift heavy weights without the risk of going through the floor.

No basement? A ground level room will suffice. The garage or outbuildings such as a barn should be a last option, unless you live in an area that has great weather conditions the year-round. Otherwise, it is difficult to control humidity (your bars and weight plates will rust) and cold weather temperatures (ungloved hands could freeze to the bar) in a non-insulated, unfinished garage. Besides, isn't your car in your garage and your cow in the barn?

Inhaling gas and oil fumes during your workout can make you dizzy and weak. Not a great scenario when you have just un-racked 315 pounds.

Maximizing workout capability in small spaces

The room—The room I use is 12 feet 8 inches x 14 feet 6 inches (184 square feet). Weight plates, bars, and accessories are stored in an area that is 3 feet 5 inches x 5 feet 5 inches (18 square feet).

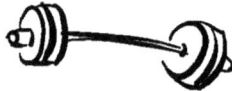

Here is how I have laid out the gym.

Sample Gym Layout

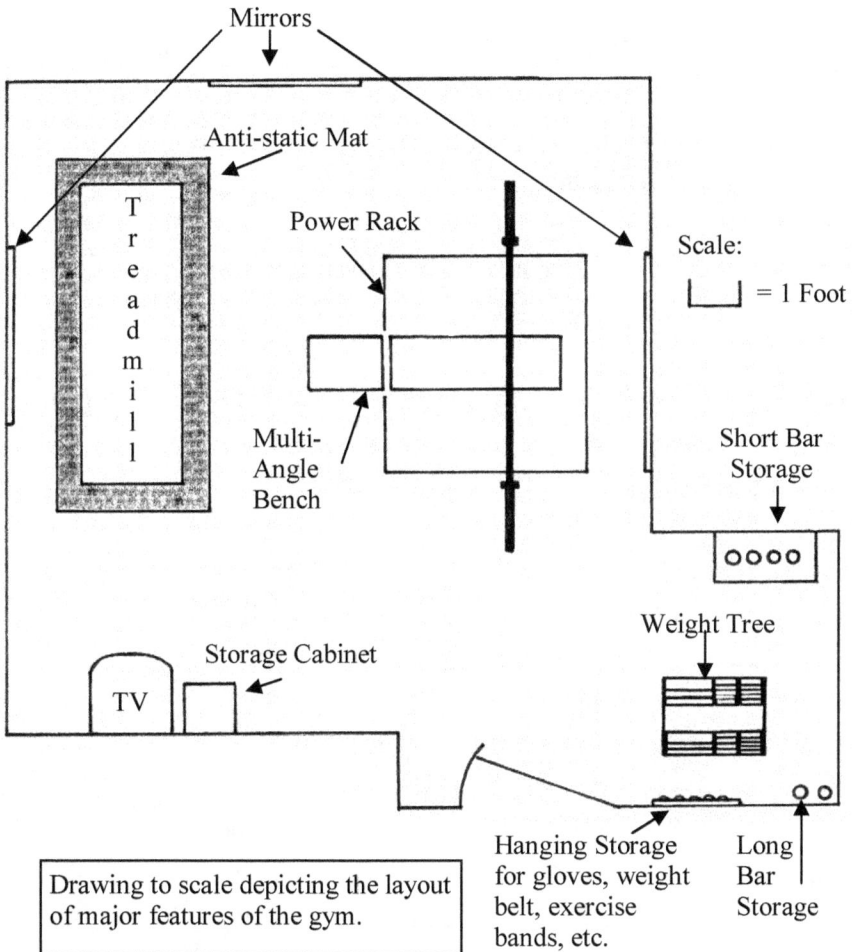

Mirrors

Anti-static Mat

Power Rack

Scale:

☐ = 1 Foot

T
r
e
a
d
m
i
l
l

Multi-
Angle
Bench

Short Bar
Storage

Weight Tree

Storage Cabinet

TV

Drawing to scale depicting the layout of major features of the gym.

Hanging Storage for gloves, weight belt, exercise bands, etc.

Long Bar Storage

The power rack is 3 feet 6 inches from the wall on the side where I load the weight. The rack is 1 foot 4 inches from the other wall so that I can enter the rack from the front or back.

There are 3 feet 7 inches between the rack and the treadmill. In this space I jump rope, do seated and standing dumbbell exercises, standing barbell presses, calisthenics, stretching, exercise ball work, and so on.

The weight tree has comfortable distances around it. I have no problems getting the weight plates I need.

Tip—Turn the 25- and 45-pound plates such that the plate's lip (rim) faces out. This affords a better grip area when pulling the plate from the weight tree.

Ceiling height—You will need a ceiling height of at least 8 feet. You do not want to put the weights through your ceiling while doing standing overhead presses.

Soundproofing—I am a very quiet lifter. All you will hear when I lift is the soft clink of one weight against its neighbor. If your lifting sessions sound akin to a demolition crew hard at work, consider adding some sound dampening materials to your gym walls. Your family members, duplex, and apartment neighbors will thank you. (On the internet search, "sound proofing materials" or "soundproofing materials" to find appropriate materials.)

Lighting—I have worked out in a place where the sole source of light was one naked incandescent bulb dangling from the ceiling. I paid $3 for the privilege.

Now I have four sets of two fluorescent light tubes illuminating my gym. Increased lighting increases gym safety. Lighting makes a world of difference as to how well a workout session goes. A dim room can sap strength, while a bright room can energize.

Room color—Lighter colors will make the gym seem brighter and larger.

Receiving equipment

Save yourself some time and frustration. Inspect all packages and their contents for damage upon delivery. The inspection is best done while the delivery person is present as a witness. If you do not do so, you may have problems getting an exchange or refund on damaged equipment.

With any piece of equipment you get, read the enclosed instruction booklets and sheets. Do this before attempting assembly or use.

Check the parts against the parts list. Make sure you have all of the required bolts, nuts, washers, screws, and other small pieces.

Find out what tools you will need before you begin.

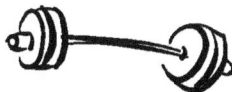

SMALL GYM BIG WORKOUTS

4

OUTFITTING YOUR GYM

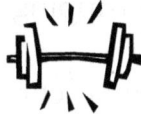

Flooring options

There are 4 feet x 6 feet x ½ inch black rubber mats covering my concrete gym floor. Each mat weighs 90 pounds. Thick rubber mats are hard to beat in terms of durability. The mats protect the concrete, the weight plates, and other equipment from damage. The rubber flooring absorbs some of the shock when placing weights on the floor. The mats are made from recycled auto tires. They give me an even, non-slip workout surface.

I purchased smooth-edged matting as opposed to the interlocking type. The interlocking matting is a staple in military gyms. However, the interlocking edges inevitably buckle and become major tripping hazards.

The two problems you may encounter with the smooth-edged matting are the sides don't square to one another, and the mats scoot away from each other over time. A utility knife and some diligent cutting will solve the first problem. Repositioning the mats every now and then will take care of the second dilemma.

If you can, get your rubber flooring several weeks before you get the rest of your equipment. This will allow you to lay the flooring out and let it 'air', preferably in a garage, outbuilding, or outside before placing the flooring in its final place. I noticed a strong aroma (petroleum?) emanating from my newly purchased mats after they were placed in my gym. It took weeks for the scent to dissipate.

Don't bother installing carpet in your gym. Several sweat-dripping workouts will leave your floor sour-smelling, stained, and mildewed.

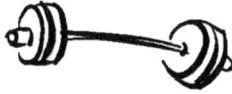

Mirror, mirror on the wall...

Mirror options

Mirrors are important parts of my gym, not for the sake of bolstering vanity, (well...maybe) but for checking progress and form. It helps to be able to see the muscles working and ensure that I am maintaining the strictest posture for the exercise.

Mirrors reflect light, thus making the room seem larger and brighter.

Three types of mirror are:
- A glass mirror with a silver-sprayed backing.
- Plexiglass™ backed with silver spray or silver sheeting.
- Highly reflective Mylar™ sheeting.

The advantages of glass mirrors are:
- They are long-lasting.
- They are highly reflective.
- They give a very clear reflection of objects.
- They are easy to clean and keep scratch free.
- They do not warp.

The disadvantages of glass mirrors are:
- They are heavy and require substantial anchoring when hung on walls.
- They can be expensive.
- They must be handled with care or cuts may result.
- They can chip, break, and shatter.

If you decide to get a glass mirror be sure to mount it high enough such that a bar loaded with 45 lb. weights will not roll into it. This, I am ashamed to say, happened to me at a military gym. I had just finished bent-over rows. I hadn't noticed the floor was slightly slanted towards the mirror. The mirror shattered, its glass shards covering a surprisingly large area. Though greatly embarrassed, I did not have seven years of bad luck. On the contrary, I did not even have to pay for the replacement mirror. Thanks, Uncle Sam!

The advantages of Plexiglas™ mirrors are:
- They are light in weight.
- They are generally less expensive than glass mirrors.
- They can be cut easily to different sizes by using a fine-tooth saw.
- They do not chip or shatter like glass mirrors.

The disadvantages of Plexiglas™ mirrors are:
- They scratch easily when you attempt to clean them.
- You will see a warped image if the wall behind the mirror is not absolutely flat.
- They will eventually yellow and become cloudy.
- Impact with a weight could crack this type of mirror.

The advantages of Mylar™ as mirrors are:
- They will be the lightest mirrors you can get.
- They are inexpensive when compared to glass or Plexiglas™ mirrors.
- They are easy to transport.
- Using scissors, they can be cut from rolls into varied lengths.
- They will not chip, shatter, or break.
- They vary in thickness from 1 millimeter to 5 millimeters. The 5-millimeter-thick sheets are highly reflective.

The disadvantages of Mylar™ as mirrors are:
- They dent. If you run a fingernail, or anything with an edge, against the Mylar's mirrored surface an indentation will be created. You will not be able to smooth out the dents. If they annoy you, it is best to cut another piece of Mylar from the roll and try again.
- Mylar is difficult to stretch onto a frame. Rather than just stapling my Mylar to the wall of my gym, I created a frame for it. The frame is made from 1 inches x 2 inches untreated wood furring strips. The Mylar was stapled to one side of the frame and stretched and stapled to the other side. This can take a few minutes or it can be hours of fun. If the Mylar is not stretched well, the result is a warped image.

I have mirrors on 3 walls; two glass mirrors and one Mylar. Get the largest mirror you can for the space you have. At the very least, have one 6 foot x 4 foot mirror mounted on the wall.

Watch out for the fun-house type of mirrors that make you look thinner or thicker. If at all possible, go to the mirror merchant and view in person the exact mirror that you will install in your gym. Tag it or write something in your handwriting on the back of the mirror. When it arrives at your house, you will know that it is the same one. I know this may sound like a lot of legwork for a simple mirror, but it is well worth it to avoid disappointing mirror distortions.

Out of sight, but not out of mind…

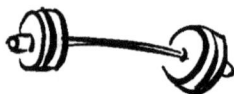

Storage space within the gym

My gym houses only the items I need to complete my workouts and some cleaning supplies. I keep everything neatly arranged so that the gym remains uncluttered.

Music CD's, DVD's, video cassette tapes, music cassette tapes, a heart rate monitor, cleaning supplies, and running shoes are stored in a 1 foot x 1 foot x 2 feet 7 inches cabinet. Within the cabinet, everything is kept organized, easily accessible, and out of sight. A compact disc radio cassette recorder sits on top of the cabinet.

All of my other workout gear is in the 3 feet 5 inches x 5 feet 5 inches (18 square feet) alcove.

A combination TV/VCR is mounted on the wall above the radio. A DVD player is mounted just below the TV/VCR. These are set up for easy viewing while I am on the treadmill.

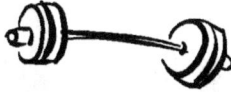

Basic equipment for your gym

Here is the basic workout equipment every home gym should have.

- A Power Rack
- A 7-foot Olympic-style weightlifting bar with a set of collars
- Two Olympic dumbbell handles with two sets of collars
- Olympic weight plates
- An Olympic weight plate tree
- A weightlifting belt
- A multi-angle (incline/flat/decline) weight bench
- Weightlifting chalk
- A treadmill with an anti-static mat placed underneath it
- A pad and pencil

Power Rack:

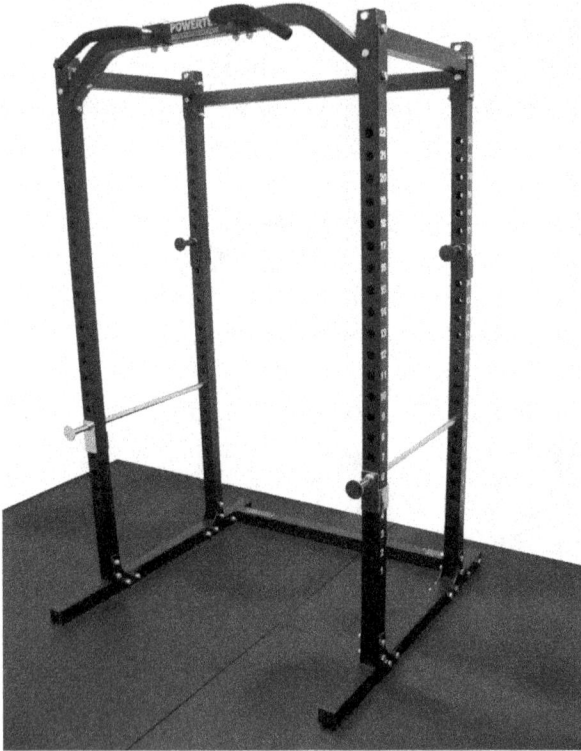

Power Rack

A Power Rack allows me to workout alone safely. After adjusting the safety rods, I can take sets to momentary muscle failure without the worry of being trapped under the weighted bar.

Powertec makes the Power Rack I have in my gym. Here is why I chose this one.

- It is built of 2-inch metal tubing.
- The safety rods and barbell rods are 1 inch thick, solid, adjustable, and will not slip out accidentally.
- There are 22 numbered adjustment holes spaced 1½ inches apart. This allows for very small, quick, and comfortable height changes.
- The weight capacity of the rack section is 1500 pounds.
- This rack does not tip in any direction when I am using heavy weights. It is very stable.
- Dip bars (rated at 400 pounds) and a dual grip chin-up bar (also rated at 400 pounds) are included in the package.
- It is roomy inside the Power Rack, so I do not feel cramped.
- When assembled, it is 4 feet 3 inches long, 4 feet 2½ inches wide, 7 feet ¾ inches high, and weighs 383 pounds.
- The price was right and it is well worth it.

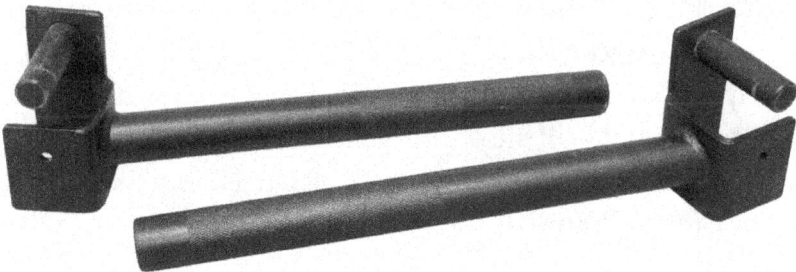

Dip bar handles

7-foot Olympic-style weightlifting bar with a set of collars:

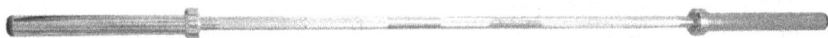

7-foot Olympic-style weightlifting bar

I have bent a lot of weightlifting bars while working out at various commercial gyms. Not on purpose. I have a great respect for another person's equipment; it is just that the bars have been weak. It is easy to find a gym that is loaded with a variety of weightlifting bars, but it is rare for a gym to have a bar rated for 800 pounds or more.

Throughout my years of lifting, my philosophy has been if there is still room on the bar it can hold more weight. All weightlifting bars do not have the same specifications. Here is what I looked for.

- A 7-foot zinc-plated weightlifting bar with a 32 millimeter diameter grip that is rated for at least 1500 pounds.
- Knurling on the bar at the left, center, and right. This rough surface where you hold the bar, allows for a surer grip. Make certain the knurling is not too sharp. Otherwise it will slice into your palm and cause injury.
- Free-spinning ends. The weight bar is less likely to roll out of your hands if the bar's ends spin freely.

Most 7-foot Olympic-style weightlifting bars weigh 45 pounds, but it varies.

26

Collars:

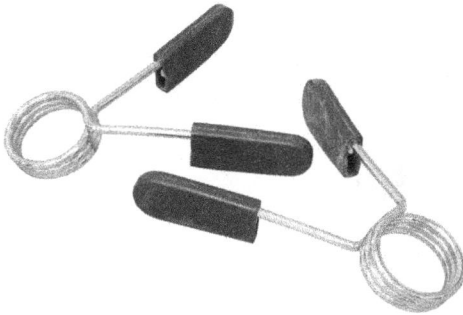

Spring-type collars

Collars, which keep the weight plates from sliding off the weightlifting bar, are not sold with a 7-foot Olympic-style bar. They will have to be purchased separately. The variety is vast.

I have chosen to use the spring-type collars on my weight bar. The spring collars are light weight. There is no twisting or turning of bolts to get the collars on or off a bar; a quick squeeze is all it takes.

Spring collars have seen me through my heaviest workouts without allowing the weights to slip off the ends of the bar.

If I find my spring collars are a bit loose on the bar, I place the round spring-side against the floor and carefully but firmly press the two handles outward and down. This tightens the spring and the spring fits the bar snugly again (provided the spring fit snugly originally).

Two Olympic dumbbell handles with two sets of collars:

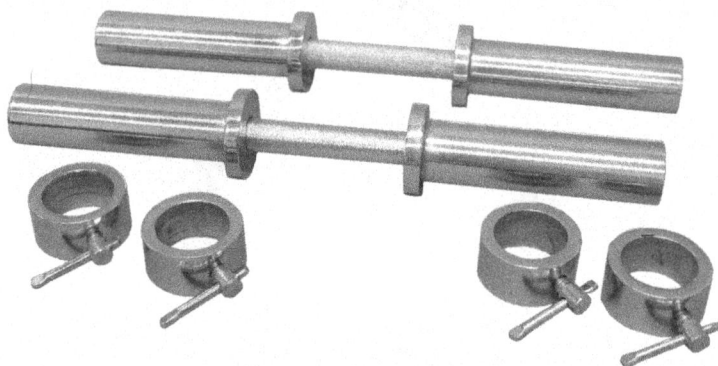

Dumbbell Handles

A crowded gym led to my first use of Olympic dumbbell handles. The dumbbells that I needed were being used, so I resorted to making my own by loading the Olympic dumbbell handles. They felt a little awkward at first, but I soon got the hang of the handles' extra length. Now I use them exclusively.

With Olympic dumbbell handles, I can go from 10 pounds to over 370 pounds per handle. These handles are great for curls, bent and upright rows, triceps, dead lifts, benching … The list goes on.

My Olympic dumbbell handles:
- Are each 20 inches long.
- Each weigh 10 pounds; 12 pounds with the collars on.
- Have a 5-inch grip area with knurling.

- Have 7-inch free-spinning ends that allow a total of 450 pounds to be loaded onto each dumbbell handle.
- Came with two collars per handle.
- Store easily out of sight.

Olympic weight plates:

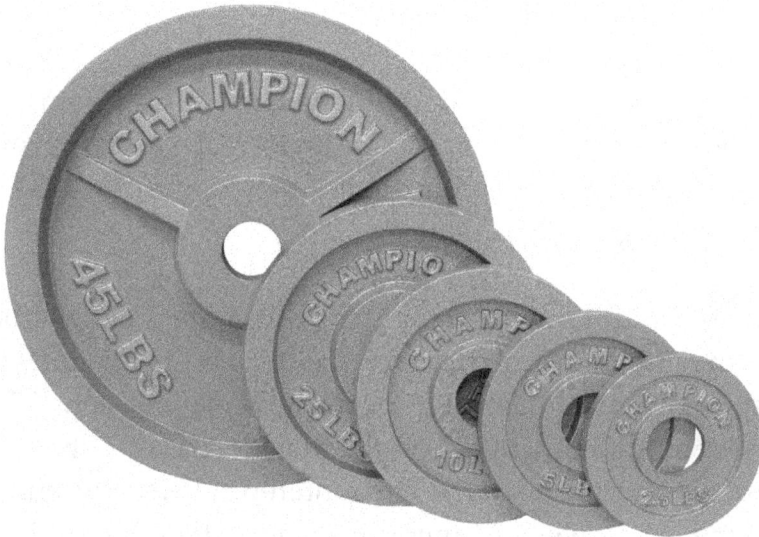

Olympic weight plates

I have a preference for free-weights. Cable weights have their place in a workout routine, but when installed in the home gym you may quickly outgrow the limited weight stack. Here is a good mix of weight plates to have.

- 4 X 2.5-pound plates (great for working through sticking points)
- 4 X 5-pound plates
- 8 X 10-pound plates

- 4 X 25-pound plates
- 45-pound plates (as many as you care to have).

When I purchased the weights for my gym, I did not get 35-pound weight plates. I've never used them much during my years of lifting. I get the equivalent weight by combining a 25-pound and 10-pound plate. By doing this I save storage space and money.

I currently keep 800 pounds of weights in my gym. If I want to go higher than 800 pounds (for shrugs) I must travel to the nearest military gym (1½ hours) or the local commercial gym (20 minutes).

I like the traditional weight plates that are solid, without the hand holes reamed out of them. The hand holes are designed to make carrying the weight plate easier. There are several different types on the market, though I have not cared for the ones I have encountered. I usually end up carrying the weight without using the hand holes. Otherwise, there is a lot of repositioning before putting the weight on the bar or back onto the weight tree. This may sound picky, but when I am thoroughly roasted at the end of a workout, the last thing I want to deal with is a fiddly weight plate. I have never dropped a weight plate, but if I ever do it will probably be the type with hand holes.

Concerning weight plate thickness, I have found there to be three overall sizes. Wide, medium, and thin flanged. The wide flanged plate is 2 inches wide, the medium is 1¼ inches wide, and the thin is about 1 inch wide. I have chosen the medium thickness. The flange's deep rim is just right for gripping and the plate is thin enough that I can get at least twenty 45-pound weight plates on my bar.

Of course I must have something to hold the weight plates when they are not in use — enter the weight plate tree.

The Olympic weight plate tree:

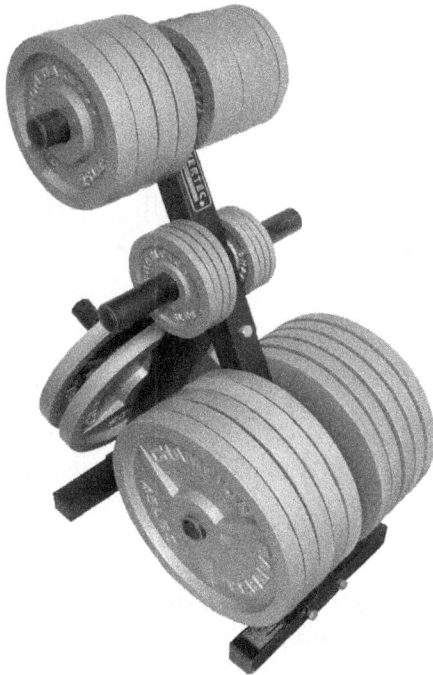

Olympic weight plate tree

Powertec makes my weight plate tree. It is constructed of 2-inch metal tubing and has seven PVC covered "weight horns" (you slide the weight plates onto the horns). It holds all of the weights I currently own and has room for more. The tree itself weighs 46 pounds. It is 28 inches long, 24 inches wide, 36 inches high, and rated for 1500 pounds.

After an exhaustive search, I found this style of weight tree to have the smallest footprint and the highest storage capacity.

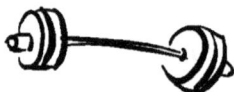

My first love is running. It is one of the reasons I'm strong but lean. I run about 40 miles a week. Running also helps keep my heart in top condition. I have heard it said that cardiovascular exercise makes a lifter small and weak. Ignore that sentiment. Watch an elite sprinter run in slow motion and marvel at the striated muscle. The heart is a muscle and it needs its fair share of exercise.

Walking is a great way to exercise too. Walking puts less stress on the knees, joints, and connective tissue than running does. This leads me to the next topic, the treadmill.

Treadmill:
A treadmill allows you to run or walk at any time of the day, regardless of the weather conditions outside. Running on a treadmill may be safer than running along the streets dodging motorists and mongrels.

Your treadmill's display panel will allow you to see at a glance:

- How fast you are running or walking.
- How long you have been at it.
- How far you have gone.
- How many calories you have burned.

Be sure to place an **anti-static mat** beneath your treadmill.

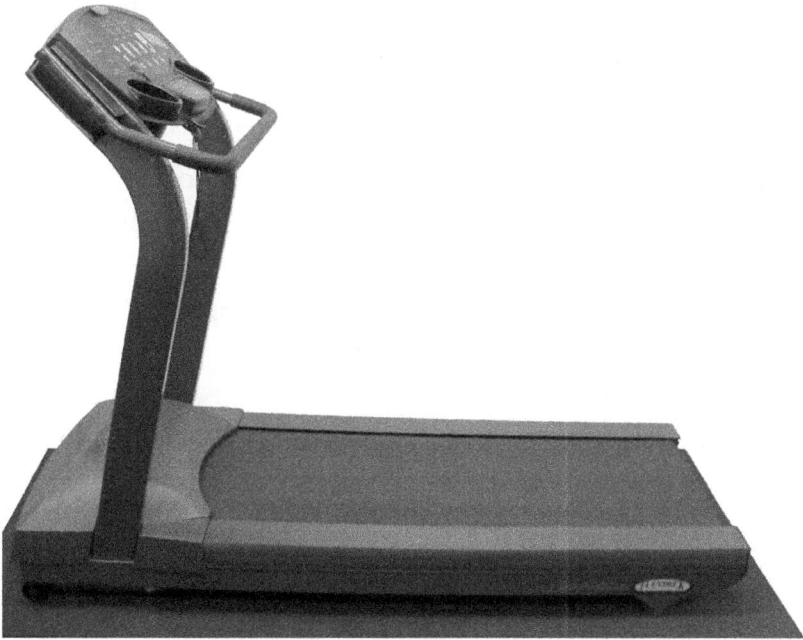

Treadmill

Choosing a treadmill

- Get a treadmill that is rated for at least a 300-pound person. A treadmill with such a rating will be sturdily constructed. If you weigh more than 300 pounds, get a treadmill with a higher weight rating.

- Make sure the bed (the part you walk or run on) is at least 50 inches long; if it is shorter your stride will suffer.
- A treadmill that is lightweight will shake around a lot when you run. Heavy treadmills shake too, but not nearly as much. Pay attention to your running style. Do not pound the treadmill when you run. If you find yourself pounding, you are better off walking. It will be better for you and your machine.

The treadmill I have is a Life Fitness T3. I have had this treadmill for years, and even though it gets four to five uses per day, it still performs as new. Here are its features:

- 7 workouts: Hill, Random, Manual, Sport training, 5k sport training, 10k sport training
- E-Z incline workouts
- Frame: 1.5 inches x 3 inches robotically welded steel frame
- 10-character LED readout
- Speed 0.5-10 mph
- Incline: 0-15%
- Power Required: 110 volts AC
- Motor system: 2.5 HP continuous duty DC MagnaDrive motor system
- Motor controller Life Fitness-designed microprocessor-based PWM controller
- Deck: ¾ inch fiberboard wax laminate, cushioned
- Deck shock absorption: FlexDeck shock absorption
- Handrail: straight front crossbar

- Belt: 54 inches long x 20 inches wide multi-ply
- Rollers: 2.0 inch precision crowned
- GoSystem™ one-touch quick start
- On-the-fly programming
- Cool down mode
- Accessory tray/reading rack
- Maximum use weight: 301 pounds
- Overall length: 72.5 inches
- Overall width: 32.25 inches
- Overall height: 55.5 inches
- Unit weight: Approximately 220 pounds
- Safety: CE, CEN, CSA, TUV, UL certified
- Warranty: Lifetime on frame and Lifespring shock absorbers
- Warranty: 15-year on motor
- Warranty: 3-year on electrical and mechanical parts
- Warranty: 1-year on labor

When you tryout treadmills, pay particular attention to the noise output. Some treadmills are noisier at the middle speeds (5.2 - 6.0), than they are at the lower or higher speeds. A loud treadmill at a showroom will sound even louder in a small space. Narrow your choices to two or three treadmills that have the features you desire and then choose the quieter treadmill, even if you have to pay a few extra dollars. During the long and short runs you will be glad you did.

Ground fault interrupter circuits are best for the treadmill and gym in general if there is a danger of moisture. Don't take the chance of sweat, sloshed water, or a sports drink shorting out your equipment and electrical circuits.

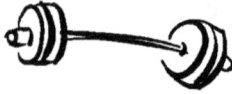

Shoes—A word on running/walking shoes. I have running/walking shoes that are used solely in the gym. By doing this I avoid getting grit and debris from the outdoors onto my treadmill's running surface, thus I greatly prolong the usefulness of the treadmill's striding belt.

Also, I replace my gym shoes every 3 months. Even though the shoes may outwardly look fine, the support system within the shoe will be in a state of decline.

Take your time when shopping for new gym shoes. No two feet are the same and choosing shoes from the large selections available in stores and on the Internet can be difficult. You could consult a shoe specialist. However, most people do not have the time or inclination to meet with a shoe specialist. You may never find shoes that provide absolute comfort and also function one hundred percent to your liking, but you can come mighty close. Following are some general guidelines to aid you.

Before shopping for shoes, it is useful to know if your feet are normal, flat, or high-arched. To determine this, wet the bottoms of your feet and then step onto a piece of paper (dark paper is best, as the wet imprint will be seen more easily). Remove your feet from the paper, and as you study the wet imprints consider this:

- "Normal" feet have moderate inward curvatures and show the forefoot and the heel connected by a wide band.
- Flat feet create imprints of the entire soles and show little or no inward curvature.
- High-arched feet show drastic inward curvature with a very thin band or no band at all connecting the forefoot and the heel.

Make sure the shoes you get have the proper arch support for your arch shape. Many shoe brands contain removable inserts. It is also possible to get custom made arch support inserts if necessary.

Here is something else to consider. When a foot strikes the ground outside heel first, it will then (generally) roll inwards until it is flat upon the ground. This normal rolling motion, called "**pronation**", absorbs shock and provides balance as you run or walk. Some people **over-pronate** (their feet roll too far inward) or **underpronate** (their feet do not roll far enough).

To find out which way your feet pronate, check the soles on the pair of shoes you wear most often. Set the pair on a shelf or table, heels towards you, so you can observe them from behind. You:

- Overpronate if your shoes show a slight inward lean. Shop for shoes that provide extra support or motion control.

- Underpronate if your shoes show a slight outward lean. Shop for shoes in the cushioning category. The cushioning shoes will allow your foot to roll closer to a "normal" pronation.
- Are neutral if there is no lean in your shoes. Shop for a neutral or stability shoe.

If you wear orthotics, have them with you when you are shopping for shoes.

Shoe prices fluctuate greatly. Watch for sales. Regardless of the price, make sure the shoes are well-made and have the features you need.

Choosing shoes—Okay, you are at the store. What do you look for in a shoe?

- Pick out a shoe you feel will look good on you. This is important. Feeling good about how you look in your workout attire can really enhance your energy level. However, the shoes must be of good quality.
- Make sure there are no obvious flaws in the footwear's construction, such as a poorly glued sole.
- With one hand grasp the shoe by the toe and with your other hand grasp the heel. Try to bend the shoe in the manner it would bend if you were walking. If it is difficult to bend, look for another shoe. Unless you require special shoes (see a foot specialist), you want shoes that will allow your foot to travel through its natural range of motion. I do not recommend very stiff shoes.

- Once you have a shoe that bends fairly easily, feel around the inside of the shoe. You are doing this to ensure there are no seams, bulges, or protrusions that might rub or snag a toenail. You want the inside of the shoe to be as smooth as possible, especially in the toe area.
- When you find a shoe that meets the above criteria, try it on.
- Your feet increase in size slightly when you run or walk, so there should be a little space between your toes and the toe of the shoe. How much space? Half an inch, or the width of your thumbnail.
- The back of the shoe should not feel too high or too low on your heel.
- If the shoe is satisfactory, examine the shoe for your other foot and try it on.
- Take an experimental walk down the aisle. If the shoe feels okay, take an experimental jog or run down the aisle. Do not be ashamed. You should feel stable in the shoes. The shoes' cushioning should be comfortable, not pillow-soft or joint-jarring hard. Your feet should not slide around inside your shoes.

Shoes tried on in a store always seem to fit differently once you get them home, so:

- Hang on to your sales slip.
- Do not throw old shoes out right away, keep them until you are sure your new pair is comfortable to use.
- Break new shoes in slowly; alternate them with your old pair for several workouts.

- Once you have broken-in your new shoes, write the current date on one of the shoes. This is so you remember when your shoes should be replaced.

I cannot stress enough the importance of a well-made and well-fitting pair of shoes. One workout in a cheap, ill-fitting pair could mean a week or more of recovery for your feet.

Socks—Wear the same type of socks you will run or walk in when trying on your shoes. Thick socks will add to the comfort of wearing the shoes. Take new socks if possible, not the threadbare "comfy" socks with the holes in them.

Weightlifting Belt:

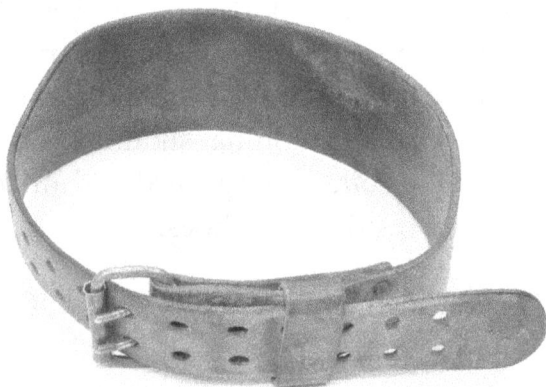

Weightlifting Belt

I am using the same sweat-stained leather weightlifting belt I have had for almost 20 years. I mention this so you will know that once you buy a good belt, you probably will not have to buy another. Weightlifting belts are essential in the gym. Mainly they:

- Help support the spine.
- Help hold the midsection in place, thus reducing the chance of a hernia.
- Help you maintain proper lifting form.

Putting on a well-made, proper-fitting, and comfortable weightlifting belt can make you feel stronger psychologically. Try it; you will see what I mean.

A multi-angle (incline/flat/decline) weight bench:

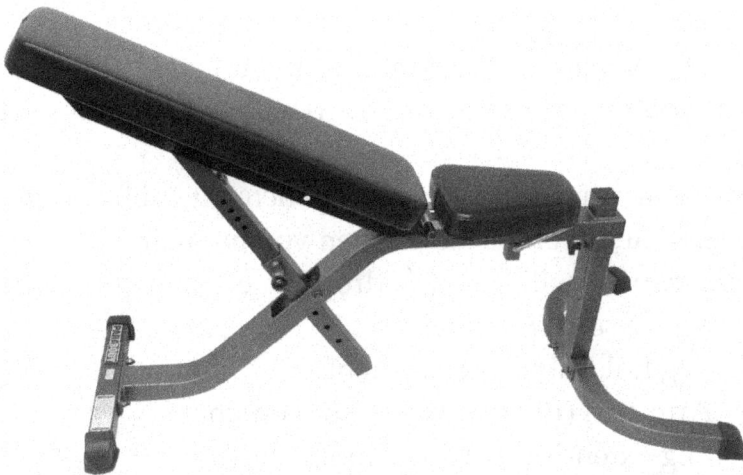

A multi-angle (incline/flat/decline) weight bench

I recommend you get only one weight bench, one capable of multi-angle adjustment.

A multi-angle bench:

- Eliminates the need for three separate benches.
- Provides varied range of adjustments.
- Is truly space-saving.

The weight bench I have is a Parabody 874 multi-angle bench. This is one solid weight bench.

- The frame of the bench is of heavy-duty steel construction.
- The padded parts are constructed of black naugahyde® (a vinyl-coated fabric) over 1⅞ inch-thick foam padding and ⅝ inch-thick plywood.
- It has a pull-pin for adjusting the seat back. You can pop it into any of the ten holes that go from the decline position to an upright shoulder press position.
- The front part of the seat can be adjusted upward, so that you do not slide from the bench when doing incline work.
- This is a very sturdy weight bench. It will not wiggle around and feel unstable when you are using it.
- The bench will accept drop-in attachment options. These are sold separately:
  - Leg hold-down attachment
  - Arm curl (Preacher curl) attachment
  - Leg extension/curl attachment
  - Lat/low row attachment (You will be hard-pressed to find it though.)

This bench weighs about 70 pounds.

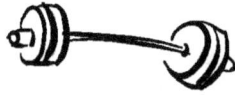

I am always a little bit nervous when I am visiting a gym that is new to me. I worry that there will either be no chalk station or a ruling outlawing the use of chalk (I usually carry my own to the gyms). Chalk is as important to me as my weightlifting belt. I generally do not have a good work-out without both of them. So this brings us to the next topic, which is about…what else? Chalk.

Weightlifting Chalk:

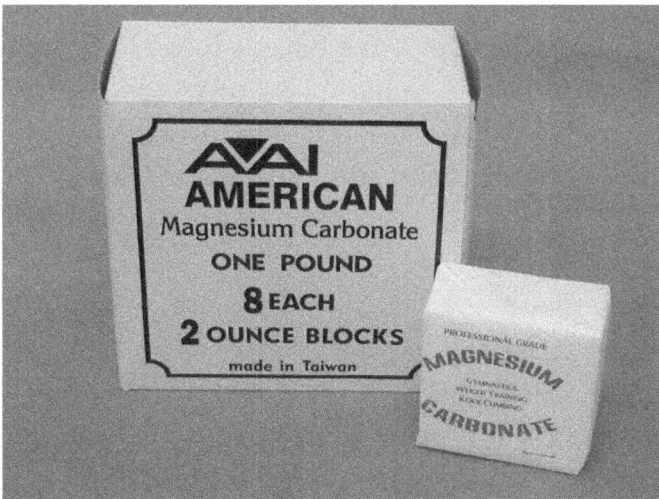

Weightlifting Chalk

I choose magnesium carbonate as my chalk. When using this type of chalk, I have never had a bar slip from my grip. I apply a light dusting before each set.

I recommend the 2-ounce block magnesium carbonate. The block allows for better control when applying the chalk. A 1-pound box containing eight 2-ounce blocks will ensure you always have chalk on hand.

I keep my chalk block in a one-quart plastic food storage container, to keep the block from being crushed. The storage container also doubles as a portable chalk station.

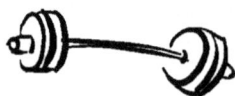

Optional workout equipment

Here are items outside of the basic equipment that can add variety, comfort, and isolation exercises to your workout. Some of the items are designed to protect your precious gym equipment from abrasion.

- Jump rope
- Exercise mat
- Olympic curl bar
- Olympic loading pin with heavy-duty carabiner
- Cable handle and small snap clip
- Leg extension attachment and Olympic sleeve adaptor
- Dip belt
- Head/neck strap
- Resistance bands
- Exercise ball
- Pushup handles
- Jerk boxes

- Punching bag
- Bag gloves, boxing gloves, and hand wraps
- Speed bag, speed bag platform, and an air pump with needle
- Barbell and Power Rack protector wraps
- 2 pound and 3 pound dumbbell sets
- Auto tire chock block

Jump rope:

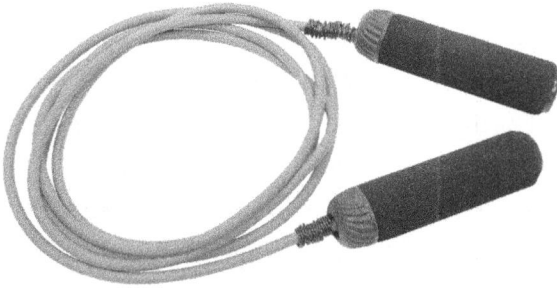

Jump rope

A jump rope is a handy, inexpensive, easily transportable alternative to other types of aerobic exercise. It's also fun to use. There are three basic types of jump ropes; cotton, synthetic, and leather. They are all available in differing lengths. They all have advantages and drawbacks.

- **Cotton**—A jump rope made of cotton is the type that you may have used as a child in the schoolyard. They have a low "ouch" factor when you flub a jump, which causes the rope to hit you in the back. Even so, I would not recommend buying a rope of this type for your gym. It is too light weight and normally has two handles that do not allow smooth turning of the rope.

- **Synthetic**—A middle-of-the-road rope is one that is synthetic. I currently use a synthetic jump rope. It has a good weight that is conducive to fluid revolutions. The handles are plastic with a neoprene foam grip.

    The problem with this type of rope is with the plastic joint that actually holds the rope. It has a sharp edge that eventually cuts through the rope. I have already had to repair mine twice. When the rope is again cut, as I know it will be, I'll upgrade to a leather rope.

- **Leather**—I think the-top-of-the-line rope is the leather rope with metal ball bearings in wooden handles. The metal ball bearings allow smooth-as-silk rotations. The leather lasts for years. The rope can be made heavier by adding moisture to the leather, although this may increase the rate of leather deterioration. There is a drawback to this type of rope. It is made evident when you flub a jump, and the rope flogs you in the back. Ooohh, Nelly!

Exercise Mat:

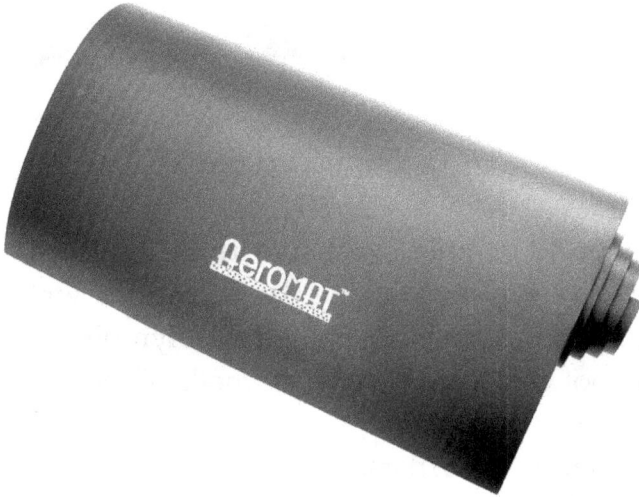

Exercise Mat

Rather than just laying a towel on the floor, lay down an exercise mat. Exercise mats are designed to cushion the bony areas of the body like the knees, elbows, and spine.

All mats do not provide the same level of performance. Get a mat that will:

- Not absorb perspiration or cleaning fluids.
- Provide you the level of cushioning you desire.
- Be long enough and wide enough for your needs.
- Be easy to roll or fold and store away.
- Not cause an allergic reaction. Make sure you know what materials were used in the mat's construction.

Olympic curl bar:

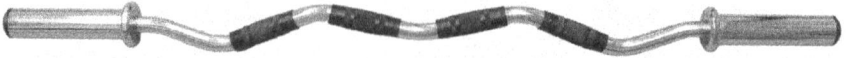

Olympic curl bar

The 22-pound Olympic curl bar with its patented Tri-Grip design allows you to grip the bar at various wrist angles. Varied grip is only one advantage an Olympic curl bar has over a 7-foot straight Olympic barbell. Other advantages are:

- It is easier on the wrists.
- The curl bar is shorter than a barbell.
- It is easier to balance.
- It is easier to load and unload weight plates.
- It imparts a great psychological motivation factor. When you see two 45-pound plates on an Olympic curl bar, it looks like a lot of weight. It is a lot of weight (110 pounds), but not as much as it would be if the two 45's were on a straight Olympic barbell (135 pounds).

There are exercises that are a lot more comfortable to do when done with a curl bar.

- Upright rows
- Close-grip bench press (The curl bar is too short to take advantage of the Power Rack's safety rods, so have someone spot you when you do this exercise.)
- Over-head triceps extensions

- Lying triceps extension
- Biceps curls
- Reverse curls
- Close-grip curls

Collars are not normally included in the price of an Olympic curl bar.

Olympic plate-loading pin with heavy-duty carabiner (D-ring clip):

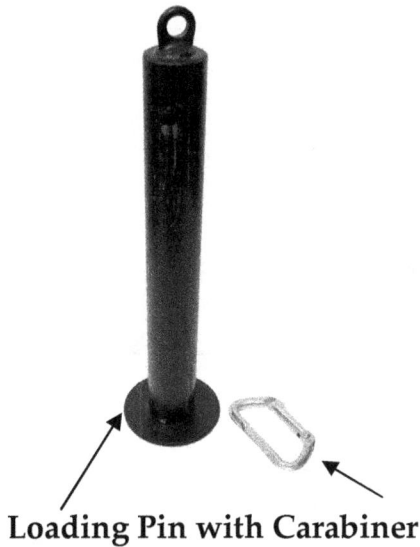

Loading Pin with Carabiner

This is a versatile tool for upper and lower body exercises. Use in conjunction with:

- A dipping belt for regular dips and hip squats.
- A head strap for working the neck.
- A cable handle for one-handed deadlifts.
- A cable bar for close-grip bent-over rows.
- A wrist roller for working the forearms.

49

The Olympic plate-loading pin:

- Is 15 inches long.
- Weighs 5 pounds.
- Has room for twelve 45-pound Olympic weight plates.

The heavy-duty carabiner (D-ring):

Is rated to hold 6000 pounds.

Tip — When loading the plates onto the Olympic loading pin, use the 2.5-pound plates as spacers. By doing this you will not smash fingers when putting weight plates onto the pin. The spacers also make it easier to get fingers under the weight plates for their removal.

Cable handle and small snap clip:

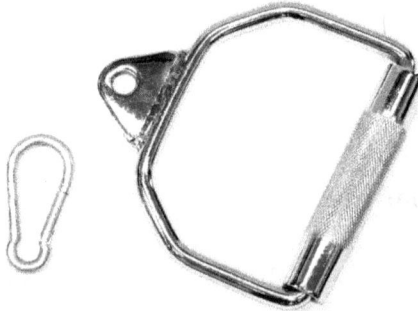

Cable handle and small snap clip

- The cable handle and small snap clip are used in conjunction with the Olympic loading pin.
- The handle weighs 2 pounds.
- It has knurling on the free-spinning grip.

Because the weight is in a straight line, you don't have to concentrate on balancing the weight when doing:

- One handed deadlifts.
- One arm reverse curls.
- One arm front and side laterals.
- One arm biceps curls.
- One arm forearm curls.

Leg extension attachment and Olympic sleeve adaptor:

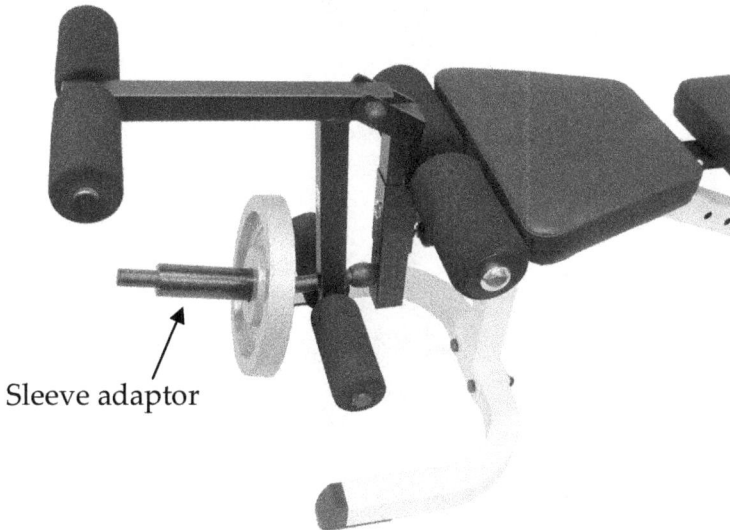

Sleeve adaptor

Leg extension attachment and Olympic sleeve adaptor

Most multi-angle weight lifting benches allow for the option of attaching a leg development attachment. Make sure you get the attachment that is specifically meant for the brand name bench you have. If you have a Parabody bench, get the Parabody attachment. This is important, because the layout of cushions for behind the knee vary from one bench manufacturer to another.

The leg development attachment will allow you to isolate:

- Quadriceps.
- Hamstrings.

Olympic sleeve adaptor:

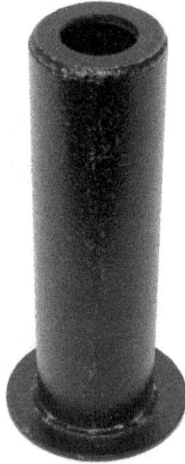

Olympic sleeve adaptor

In order to use Olympic weight plates with the leg development attachment, you will need an Olympic sleeve adaptor. Generally, any brand of Olympic sleeve adaptor will do. The sleeves vary in length, material construction, and price.

I have a **Kamway** Olympic sleeve adaptor. It is:

- Constructed from metal with a baked on black enamel paint.
- 7 inches long.
- Capable of holding five 45-pound Olympic weight plates.

Weights must be added to the opposite end of the weight bench for counterbalance.

Dip belt:

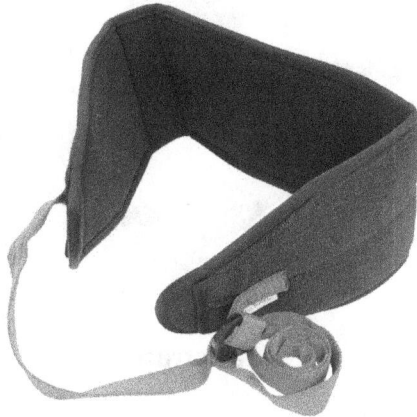

Dip Belt

The dip belt allows you to do weighted: dips, chin-ups, squats, and calves. The dip belt I have is a **De Rigeur Dipping Belt.** It is:

- The most comfortable dip belt I have ever used.
- 2 pounds in weight.

- Made of tough, woven nylon webbing on the outside. A soft, brushed tricot lining covers padding on the inside.
- Equipped with a thick, enameled buckle through which I double loop the strap that holds the weight plate's weight. The strap is also made of durable nylon.
- Fully adjustable, one size fits all.
- Capable of holding 1000 pounds.

Headstrap:

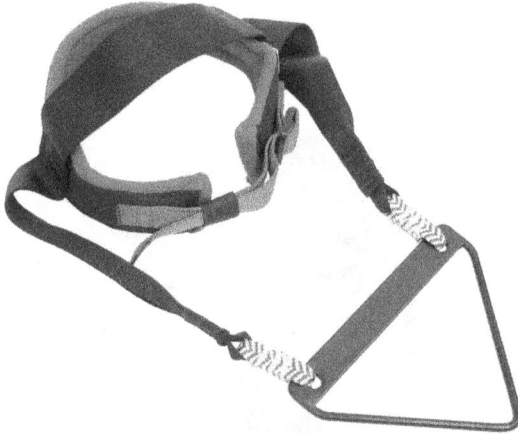

Headstrap

A time may come when you will want to strengthen your neck muscles. When that time comes, reach for the **'Headstrap Fit For Hercules™'**. This headstrap:

- Is tops for neck isolation exercises.
- Is the most comfortable headstrap I have ever used.
- Does not squeeze the head when weight is added.
- Is fully adjustable.

- Will fit most head sizes.
- Can be used with or without the loading pin and heavy-duty carabiner (D-ring clip).
- Weighs 2 pounds.
- Holds hundreds of pounds.

The neck is usually the weakest link in a body's musculature, so be extremely careful and patient when doing neck exercises.

Resistance bands:

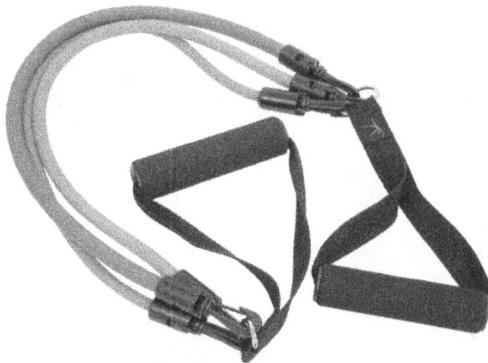

Resistance bands

Beginners as well as long-time lifters can benefit from the use of resistance bands. Resistance bands:

- Are a great tool to use for building core strength. Core strength relates to how strong the muscles of your abdomen, waist, and lower back are. A strong core is important for keeping your spine in alignment, which helps you avoid back pain and problems.

- Can be used for adductor and abductor exercises. Just loop one end of the band around your leg or ankle, and the other end to a sturdy stationary object like your Power Rack. Move your leg away from the center of your body for abductor work (outer thigh), and toward the center for adductor work (inner thigh).
- Are lightweight and easily transported; thus allowing you to do a host of exercises (curls, triceps, squats, abs, rotator cuff, etc.) almost anywhere.

Exercise ball (a.k.a. Stability ball):

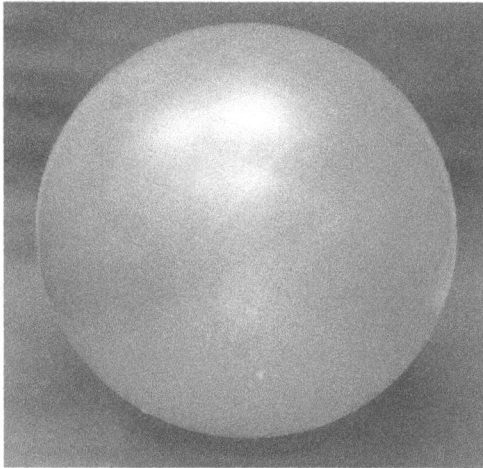

Exercise ball

The exercise ball is a good piece of equipment for maintaining or rehabilitating spine health. It's also good for abdominal exercises. It helps by bringing the stabilizer muscles into play and, as a result, strengthens the body's core.

An air pump should be included in the exercise ball's purchase price; but check to make sure.

Pushup handles:

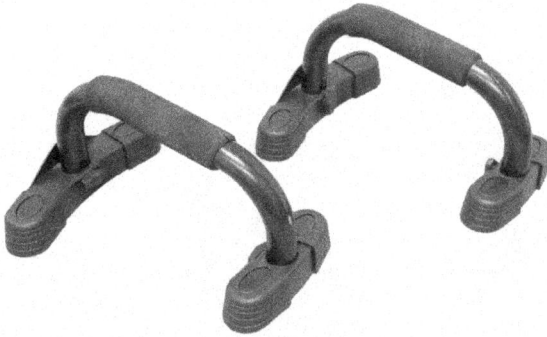

Pushup handles

Pushups are excellent for building upper body strength without the use of additional weights. They are also good for your stabilizer muscles.

Many organizations, the military tops the list, use the maximum number of pushups a person can do in the assessment of the person's upper body strength and fitness level. Whenever possible, use pushup handles when doing pushups. Pushup handles:

- Allow the wrists to be in a straight, strong, and comfortable knuckle-down position.
- Allow for a deep stretch at the bottom of the pushup movement.
- Are portable.
- Are inexpensive.

Doing pushups until momentary muscle failure is the only way I have found to increase the number of pushups I am able to do.

Jerk or Pulling boxes:

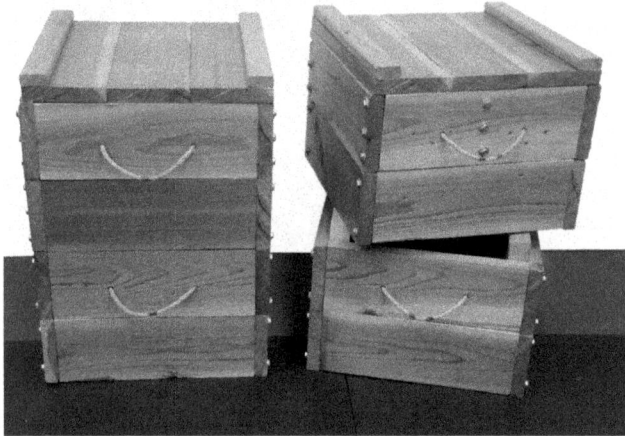

Jerk or Pulling boxes

Jerk or Pulling boxes are usually wooden boxes that allow you to situate weights at varying heights from the floor. Since you build them, you can make them taller or shorter to comfortably fit your height. Pulling boxes are versatile and allow you to:

- Platform weights 12 or 24 inches off the floor for heavy dumbbell work.
- Isolate muscle groups.
- Work on blasting through sticking points.
- Save wear and tear on your back.
- Perform exercises that require the use of a sturdy box.

Punching bag:
The punching bag I have is 32 inches long, weighs 30 pounds, and was made by me. This punching bag is:

- Great for cardio sessions.
- An awesome calorie burner.
- A stress reliever.
- Also a reaction bag when bungee cords are used at the top and bottom of the bag.
- An excellent punching tool for boxing as well as martial arts.
- Inexpensive.
- As hard or soft as its maker desires.
- Not difficult to add weight to or take weight from.

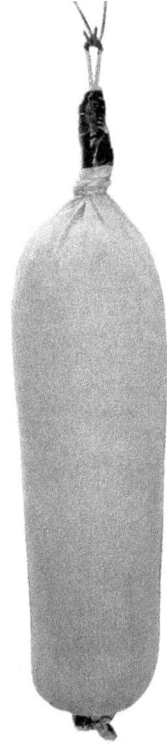

To use this bag I hang it from the front cross bar of my Power Rack using a small bungee cord. A longer bungee, which is attached to the bottom of the bag, is placed under a weight plate. This makes it akin to a 'reaction' bag, and keeps the bag from swinging around too much when it is punched.

Punching bag

Hand wraps, bag gloves, and boxing gloves:
Never punch a punching bag without first putting on hand wraps and bag gloves. Even a few moderate punches without either of these can leave your knuckles with less skin and your wrists sore.

The hand wraps:

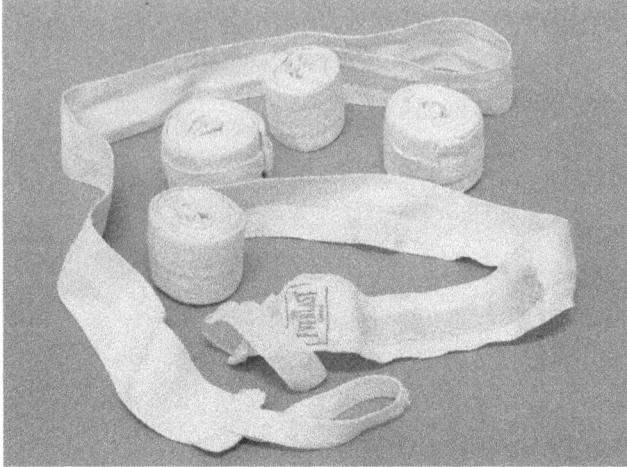

Hand wraps

- Help to stabilize your wrists.
- Help to protect your knuckles from the friction of the inside of the gloves as you work the bag.
- Aid in the protection of the small bones of your hands.
- Absorb perspiration from your hands while they are in the gloves. This helps with glove hygiene and extends the usefulness of your gloves.

Hand wraps come in varying lengths. Some examples are 195 inches for professionals, 170 inches for large hands, 120 inches for medium hands, and 108 inches for small hands.

The shorter hand wraps can be found at most department stores. The longer hand wraps can be found at stores specializing in boxing or martial arts equipment. All sizes can be found on the Internet.

The boxing gloves and bag gloves:

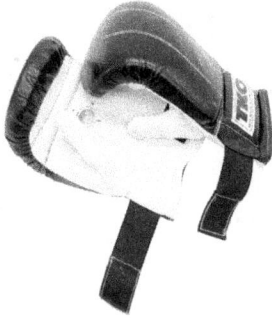

Boxing gloves   **Bag gloves**

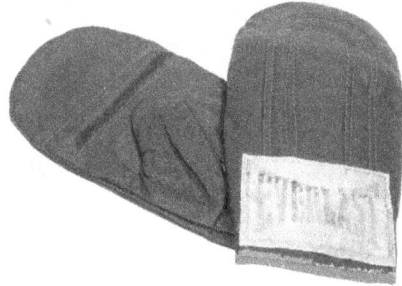

- Are generally made of polyurethane or leather. Polyurethane gloves tend to be cheaper than leather gloves. However, leather gloves are tougher and are designed to endure heavy use.
- Fit snugly over your wrapped hands.
- Protect your hands by providing some cushioning.
- Differ in size and weight. Boxing gloves (a.k.a. sparring gloves) have more padding, are heavier, and give more protection than bag gloves (a.k.a. bag mitts).
- Are highly recommended if you plan to punch a bag.

It is a joy to work the bag in gloves that fit well and a misery if the gloves are ill fitting.

- If you can, buy your gloves locally and try the gloves on before you purchase them.
- Take your hand wraps with you and wrap your hands before putting on the gloves.
- Your hands should not slide around in the gloves.
- The gloves should be snug but not overly tight.

- Make sure the gloves have Velcro, not strings, as you will not be able to tie the strings yourself.
- Make certain the gloves are right for you before you walk out of the store.

Mail-ordered boxing gloves usually cannot be returned if you have ordered the wrong size by mistake. When you are buying your gloves, make sure you understand the merchant's return policy. Keep your receipt.

Speed bag platform, speed bag, air pump with needle:

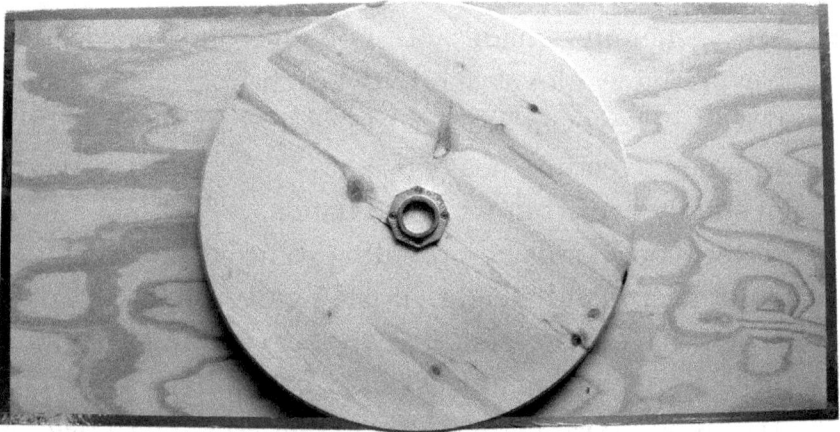

Speed bag platform

The speed bag platform in this book was designed by me to be used in conjunction with the Power Rack.

- The materials list is inexpensive when compared to a sturdy mail-ordered model.
- Constructing the platform is easy.

- The finished product is much better than the freestanding models you will find at department stores. Don't buy those. They will only disappoint you.
- The platform is easy to put up or take down, when using the homemade PVC assisting hooks.
- I have used this workout after workout with outstanding results.

The only drawback, if there is one, is the platform is set at a fixed height. People 5 feet 5 inches to 6 feet 2 inches should have no problem using it. Taller people? I can't say. Shorter people may need to stand on a platform.

Speed bag:

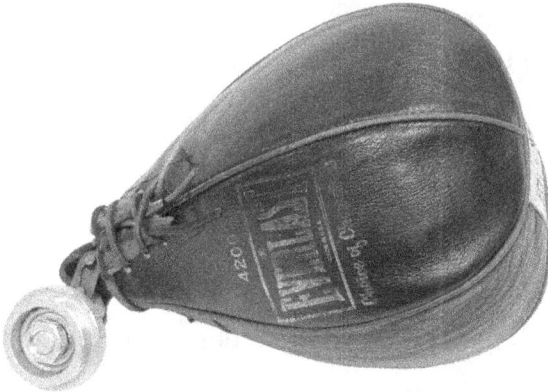

Speed bag

A speed bag:

- Is a terrific cardio tool.
- Improves reflexes.
- Strengthens muscles.

- Works the shoulders and upper back.
- Helps build upper body stamina.
- Is a hand and eye coordination enhancer.
- Increases punching speed for martial arts and boxing.
- Can be used to practice complex rhythms and punching combinations.
- Is just plain fun to use.

Speed bags come in different sizes; large, medium, and small. The smaller the bag, the faster it rebounds when it is struck. The bag I have is a 9 inches x 6 inches Everlast 4200 Sonic. It is classified as a small-sized bag with a fast rebound; and is generally not recommended for beginners. If you are a beginner, you can slow the bag's rebound by letting a little air out of the bag. Don't let so much air out that the bag shows wrinkles.

As your coordination increases, add a little more air to the bag. Keep doing this as you progress, but never pump the bag beyond its recommended air pressure. You may cause injury to your hands or the bag.

Most speed bags are deflated when you purchase them, so have an air pump and 'inflation needle' handy. To avoid damaging the internal bladder, be sure to moisten the needle before inserting it into the bottom of speed bag.

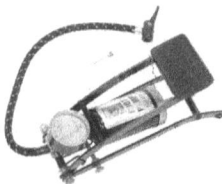

Air pump with needle

Barbell and Power Rack protector wraps:

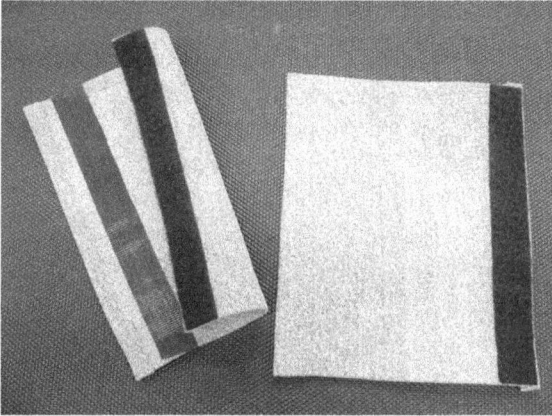

Barbell and Power Rack protector wraps

These are wraps that go around the knurling at both ends of the weight bar. They:

- Extend the usefulness of your equipment.
- Create a barrier against friction between the weight bar and Power Rack.
- Prevent the creation of iron filings that might get into your eye or under your skin.
- Keep the rack's paint from being scratched off, thus avoiding rust issues.
- Dampen sound.
- Are quick and easy to put on or take off.
- Are simple and inexpensive to make.

2-pound and 3-pound dumbbell sets:

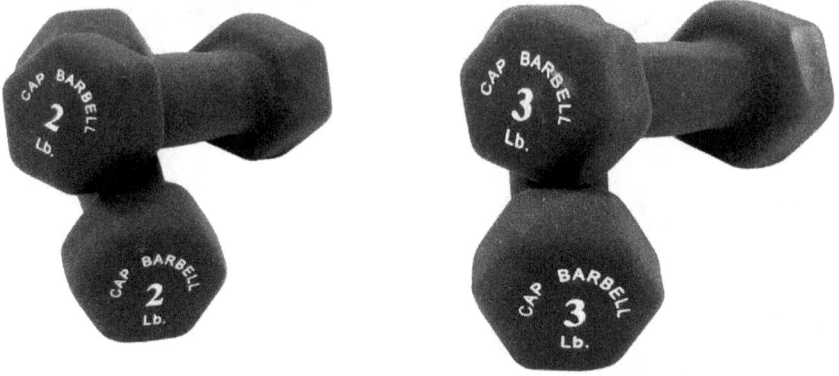

2-pound and 3-pound dumbbell sets

Light dumbbells, one 2-pound pair and one 3-pound pair, are useful for:
- Bumping up the number of calories you burn during a treadmill session.
- Building upper body strength and stamina without bulking up.
- Gently warming up the shoulders before doing more strenuous exercises.

The dumbbells I have are metal and enamel coated. However, you may opt to get the dumbbells that sport a soft, colorful synthetic covering. The synthetic covering will absorb some moisture, but this should not cause you to lose your grip.

Auto tire chock block:

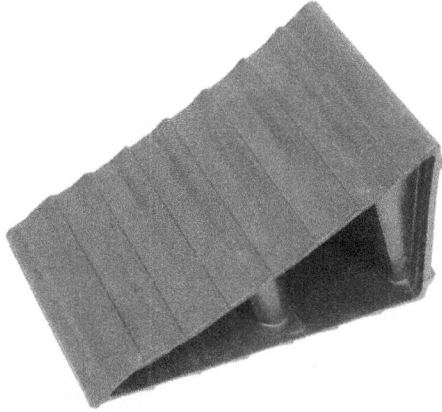

Auto tire chock block

"Okay, Mack," you say, "what is an auto tire chock block doing in your gym?" Well, I have found it to be an excellent tool to use for stretching my Achilles tendons and calves. The chock block is:

- Not scooting around when I am using it.
- Angled just right for a good stretch.
- Lightweight but durable plastic.
- Inexpensive.
- Very transportable. On the occasions when I go abroad, I can take it with me to use before and after workouts.

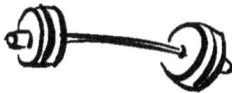

Nice-to-have accessories

- Weight plate spacer
- Room air filter
- Multi-media station
- Dip bars, dumbbell handles, and loading pin organizer

Weight plate spacer:
Whenever I have worked out in a gym, be it military or commercial, I could not fail to notice several of my fellow gym-rats sporting purple fingernails. It was the tell-tale sign that they had mashed their fingers between two weight plates. Since the only things I like mashed are my potatoes, I use weight plate spacers on the weight tree in my gym.

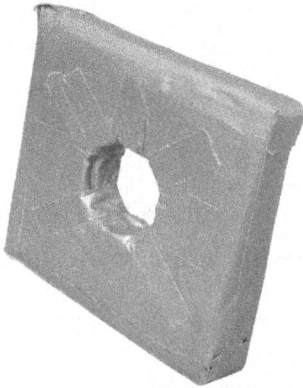

Weight plate spacers:

- Create finger space between weight plates.
- Allow easier weight plate retrieval and replacement.
- Are inexpensive and easy to make.

Weight plate spacer

Room air filter:

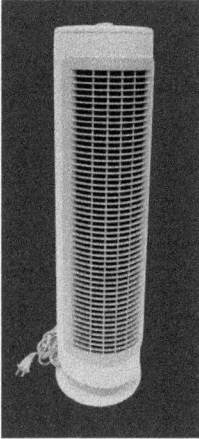

Room air filter

A room air filter will help improve the air quality in your gym. The filter I have is a streamlined tower-type. It only uses a little energy, so I keep it turned on all the time. I know it is removing dust particles from the air, because I have had to change the filter several times. Even so, I still find that a complete manual room dusting is needed each week. Dust seems to appear as if by magic. The air filter helps, but alone it will not keep your gym 100% dust free.

Multi-media station:

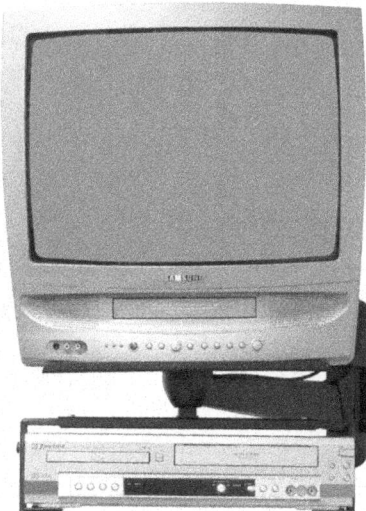

Multi-media station

Having a television and DVD player included in a multi-media station can help keep you motivated during your workouts. You will be able to listen to your desired music or watch your favorite programs while you are on your treadmill. A multi-media station bids boredom bye-bye. Pop in a DVD on physics and exercise your brain as well as your muscles.

Dip bars, dumbbell handles, and loading pin organizer:

Your gym can become cluttered in a hurry if you have no way to organize your dip bars, dumbbell handles, and loading pin. Don't just stack them in a corner, store them in an easy-to-make organizer. Using the organizer will keep your equipment handy and out of your way.

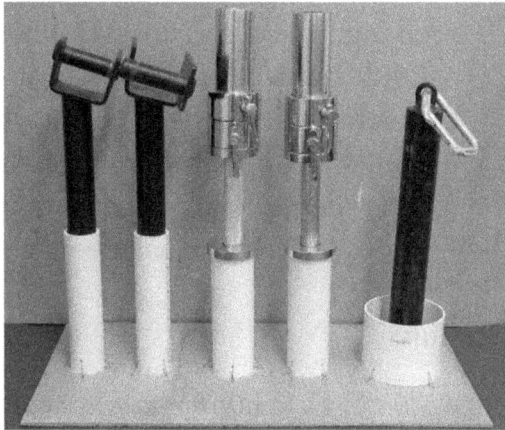

Dip bars, dumbbell handles, and loading pin organizer

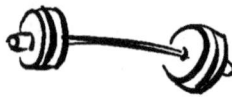

Where to buy gym equipment

If you are buying on the Internet, make sure you are buying from a reputable company. Check online reviews concerning the company's services and customer satisfaction. If anything seems shady or makes you feel uneasy about the company, look someplace else.

I have purchased many items from **Fitness Resource**. They have excellent equipment and service. They have showrooms where you can see and tryout the equipment before you buy. Fitness Resource often runs "buy-one-get-another-something-free" sales. Check out their web site to see if there is a showroom near you.

www.fitnessresource.com

Mega Fitness is an online site that sells top-quality exercise equipment. Their selection is vast. Their prices are reasonable and on many items shipping is free.

www.megafitness.com

Amazon.com is a place you may want to look for Olympic weight plates. Weight plates are normally sold for x-number of cents per pound of weight. I have found the best price per pound at Amazon.

www.amazon.com

New and used equipment can be found in your local newspaper's classified section.

Check your phonebook for fitness equipment stores. If you find a piece of equipment you like at a local store, but the price seems high, check on the Internet for a better price. Remember to take into account the mail order shipping costs.

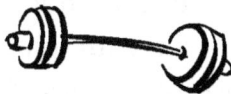

Where to get gym equipment for free

Monitor media. Listen to the radio and watch the newspaper and television for exercise equipment store specials. Sometimes stores will give you a free piece of equipment when you make a purchase. If the free equipment item is not something you want, you may be able to choose another piece of equipment of equal or lesser value in exchange. Haggle before you buy.

Convenience centers. I live in an area where I must deliver my household trash and recyclables to the local landfill myself. So this is how I discovered the landfill has a convenience center. The convenience center is a place where people can drop off unwanted but still useable items. Any item in the center is yours for free. I have seen large mirrors, treadmills, exercise bikes, a Bow flex, weight bars, cable machines, Nordic tracks, rowing machines, stair climbers, trampolines, and some Olympic weight plates (which I quickly snatched up). Anyone can take as many items as they want from the convenience center. No matter where you live, there is bound to be a landfill and convenience center not too far away. Check out this place on the weekends or when you have time—you may just find something you can use.

Offer to "equipment sit". You may know of someone who owns exercise equipment but does not use it. Make an offer to house their equipment at your place in return for the privilege of using it. Since the equipment will be a loan, he retains ownership, but eventually he may tell you to just keep it because he likes having the freed-up space.

Retirement Gifts. If you are soon to retire from your job, tell your boss to forget about giving you a golden watch for your years of diligent service, and tell him or her you would prefer a Power Rack or treadmill. Better yet ask for a Power Rack and a treadmill, you have, after all, practically thrown your back out working for the company. It is the least your boss can do.

Graduation gifts. Graduating from college? Tell your parents not to give you a new set of wheels as a graduation present. The price of gas is outrageous, driving conditions are terrible, and insurance coverage is costly. Ask your parents to outfit your home gym instead, where you can build a truly impressive set of "wheels" (legs).

Wish Lists. Give your friends, co-workers, and family a gym equipment wish list. Update it often, so if they ever decide to throw a surprise party for you they can surprise you with, say, 300 pounds worth of Olympic weight plates. In other words, something you really want. The same goes for birthday and holiday lists.

Newspapers. Scan the newspaper's classified section. You may find that some people will give you equipment for free if you will haul it away. Check for yard sales and arrive late in the day. If exercise equipment has not sold by the end of the sale, the proprietor may give it to you for free so he avoids the hassle of hauling it to the landfill.

Gymnasiums. Do you have a gym membership? If the owner of the gym is getting new equipment, ask if you can have the old equipment. The owner may be happy to let you have it, as storage space is always in short supply in gyms. Be prepared to haul it yourself.

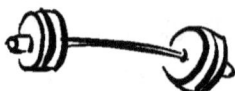

How to buy equipment

If at all possible, buy your equipment locally. This way you can inspect, touch, and even use the equipment before you purchase it. Do not abuse the merchandise (you have not paid for it yet) but run it through its paces. Make sure the equipment will perform the function or functions you want it to. Do not be shy.

Carry your **clean-soled** workout shoes with you to the showroom. You may even want to dress in sweats (clean sweats, please). Do not be ashamed or hesitant to walk or run on a prospective treadmill. Lie on the weight benches. Adjust the benches through their ranges. Heft the weight bars and choose weight plates that you can grip comfortably. Try on the weightlifting belt. Try every piece you plan to buy. Do not be afraid to ask the sales person many questions. Doing all of this will help you avoid disappointing surprises later.

Take a **tape measure** with you to the store. Feel free to measure the dimensions (height, width, and depth) of the equipment you plan to buy to ensure it will fit in your gym.

Equipment that is flimsy, poorly constructed, or made from substandard materials has no place in the home gym. Beware. Most of the so-called home gym items for sale in department stores have these undesirable features.

Get the best equipment for your money; the extensive checklist below will help ensure that you do.

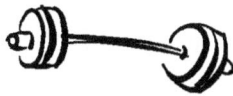

Checklists for basic equipment

Note: (I) stands for checklist information available to you when evaluating equipment on the Internet. This information is useful when you absolutely cannot be in the room with a given piece of equipment before you buy it. The absence of an (I) means you should perform the visual checks and tests in person. Copy the checklist and have it with you when making your evaluations.

Multi-angle bench:

◊ Does it adjust smoothly and easily through its full range of positions?
◊ Is the padding thick and firm?
◊ Do the parts that swivel do so smoothly?
◊ Does the bench feel sturdy? Give the bench a firm shake. If it rattles like pennies shaken in a tin can, it may have a loose bolt. Ask an employee if it can be tightened.

◊   (I) How much does the bench weigh? Make sure the bench is not too heavy for you to pick up and move about, as you will be doing this in your gym. Some benches sport wheels for easy relocating.

◊   Is the bench the right height for you? Put the bench in the flat position. Lie on it. Your feet should rest flat on the floor when you are lying 'face up' on the bench.

◊   Is the frame well welded or bolted together?

◊   Is the padding covered with a durable material (like Naugahyde), well sewn, well fitted, and firmly attached to wood under the bench's pads?

◊   Does the adjustment pin seat properly, work easily, and adjust smoothly?

◊   Is there a 'foot hold down'? If the bench has a 'foot hold down', test it to make certain it has enough padding to cushion your ankles and the backs of your knees.

◊   Is the paint chipped or scratched?

◊   Are all of the plastic caps present on the bench's feet and other openings in the bench's frame?   Caps should be new.

◊   Do you feel comfortable and stable in all positions? Physically try the bench in its upright, incline, flat, and decline positions.

◊   When the bench is in the flat or decline position, is there a gap between the bench's back and seat? The gap should not be so large as to be uncomfortable to your lower back.

◊   (I) What are the warrantee's terms and conditions?

Bars and Dumbbell Handles:

Does the bar or handle:

◊ (I) Meet your preferred load rating?
◊ Have 'free-spinning' ends that rotate smoothly?
◊ Have knurling that is not too sharp?
◊ Have chips or flakes in the finish?
◊ Have ends that are firmly bolted to the main bar?
◊ Fit comfortably in your clenched hand(s)?
◊ (I) Have sufficient length for your needs (i.e. Power Rack)?
◊ (I) Have ends long enough to take the number of 45-pound weights you wish to load?
◊ (I) Come with collars?
◊ Need an Allen wrench to periodically tighten the end bolts?
◊ (I) Have a warrantee?

Weight Plates:

◊ (I) Will the clang of weight plates as you use them in your gym create a noise issue? If so, choose rubber weights.
◊ (I) Does the weight plate's flanged rim offer a finger-hooking area for carrying the plate more easily?
◊ Are the painted or enameled plates chipped?
◊ (I) Are the plates treated against rust?
◊ Is rust evident?

◊ (I) Are the plates thin-flanged, medium-flanged, or wide-flanged?

◊ (I) Are handholds cut into plates?

Treadmill:

◊ (I) Is it rated for 300 or 400 pounds?

◊ (I) Is the motor of the continuous duty type, and at least 2.5hp?

◊ (I) Is the voltage rating 110 volts or 220 volts? Make sure it matches the voltage available in your gym area.

◊ (I) Is the deck striding area length at least 50 inches?

◊ (I) Is the stride belt multi-ply with a textured surface?

◊ (I) Is the deck cushioned?

◊ Is the deck comfortable to walk/run on?

◊ (I) What are the minimum and maximum speeds?

◊ Is the treadmill quiet, or acceptably quiet, at all speeds?

◊ (I) Will the deck incline to at least 15%?

◊ (I) Is the console easy to navigate?

◊ (I) Does the console display distance, calories burned, speed, and/or level of difficulty?

◊ (I) What is the maximum time allowed for a manual workout session?

◊ (I) Are there pre-programmed and manual workout settings?

◊ (I) Is there an emergency stop switch?

◊ (I) Is there a heart rate monitor?

◊ (I) Are there water bottle holders?

◊ (I) Is there a reading rack?

◊ (I) Is there a handrail?

◊ (I) What does the treadmill weigh?

◊ Do you need an anti-static mat?

Power Rack:

◊ (I) Is it taller than the room it will be in?

◊ (I) Is it made of steel, well welded, free of cracks, and covered with a rust barrier?

◊ (I) Are the holes for safety rods 1½ inches to 2 inches apart and numbered for easy adjusting?

◊ (I) Are there 1-inch thick safety rods that will not accidentally slip out when in use?

◊ Is the rack rickety when assembled? Test the store's model. If it is rickety in the store, it will most likely be rickety when assembled in your gym.

◊ (I) Is there a chinning bar with multiple hand grips?

◊ (I) Is there a dip station option?

◊ (I) Does the rack hold at least 300 pounds more than will be used on it? Example: If your maximum lift will be 500 pounds, the rack should be rated for no less than 800 pounds. This is a safety factor and it also takes into account your future strength increases.

◊ (I) Are the dimensions such that you have adequate room to work freely within the rack?

◊ (I) Will the Power Rack fit comfortably inside your gym? Check its dimensions to ensure it will fit into its allotted gym space.

◊ (I) Are the holds (hooks) for the barbell of a design that prevents the barbell from accidentally rolling off?

◊ (I) What are the warrantee's terms and conditions?

Weight Plate Tree:

◊ (I) Does it have sleeves for Olympic-style weight plates?

◊ (I) Is it rated for the amount of weight you wish to store?

◊ Is it well welded and/or bolted together?

◊ Does the tree have chipped enamel, rust, or flaking paint present?

◊ Are all plastic caps present and in new condition?

◊ (I) Does it meets your desired dimensions?

◊ (I) Is assembly required?

◊ (I) What are the warrantee's terms and conditions?

Weightlifting Belt:

◊ Does the belt fit around your waist?

◊ (I) Is it of a thick, durable material like leather or nylon?

◊ Does the belt fit comfortably?

◊ Is the buckle or cinching device well made?

◊ Does the buckle secure the belt around your waist

quickly and easily?
◊ Is the belt easy to remove from around your waist?

Weightlifting Chalk:

◊ (I) Is the chalk magnesium carbonate?

Once you are satisfied that the product is the right one for you, ask if the item will be going on discount soon. It never hurts to ask, and you may be pleasantly surprised.

Haggling sometimes works. You will not be able to haggle in the United States like you would if you lived overseas, but if you are willing to buy several items from the merchant, he or she may give you a nice discount.

However, locally purchased equipment does not always translate to huge savings. If the local merchant's price seems outlandishly high and the merchant is unwilling to give a discount, thank him or her kindly and look online for a cheaper price.

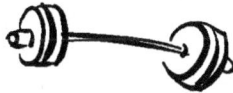

Equipment delivery versus hauling it yourself

Try to get as much equipment as you can from one place, this way you may combine the delivery to keep your delivery costs low.

Treadmill:

My treadmill was delivered already assembled. Of course I paid 50 dollars for this privilege, but I feel it was worth it. The deliverymen were employees of the place from which I bought the treadmill. They carried it into my gym, situated it exactly where I desired it, and made on-the-spot checks to ensure the treadmill worked perfectly.

If you can, have your treadmill delivered. I highly recommend delivery because:

- You will not need any tools to set it up.
- You can start using it right away.
- The striding belt's tension will have been set at the factory so you should not have to worry about slippage.
- The treadmill's weight is over two hundred pounds, including packaging, and can be awkward to move into your gym.
- The technicians will be on hand to show you how to properly operate the treadmill and answer any questions you may have. They can also immediately detect and rectify any problems with the equipment.

*Make sure you know exactly what your delivery charge entitles you to. Will you get delivered to your gym room an assembled product and an equipment check like I did? Or is delivery limited to an unassembled product placed on your doorstep? Get the facts, preferably in writing, before you pay.

Power Rack:
The Power Rack is long and it will extend past the rear bumper when placed in most passenger vehicles. This protrusion creates a safety hazard on the road. The better part of valor is to have the rack delivered.

My Power Rack arrived boxed and disassembled. Yours will too. I strongly urge you to:

- Open the box and inspect the parts and pieces while the delivery person is still present.
- Make sure you have received the proper rack.
- If needed, fill out a damage report immediately.

Hopefully you will not have any problems. I did not.

7-foot Olympic-style weightlifting bar:
Keep in mind the length of this bar. If you cannot fit it into your vehicle such that it will not eject through a rear or front windshield when you hit your brakes, have it delivered. To allow the bar to hang out of a window is not a safe option; neither is trying to secure it to the top of your car. If you must have your bar immediately, borrow your friend's pickup truck.

Olympic weight plates:

Generally, hauling weight plates in your car is not a problem. This applies to a total of 400 pounds or less. You will be able to situate this amount of weight throughout your vehicle, such that it does not flop or shift about if you have to accelerate sharply or jam on your brakes.

Do not try to haul 500 pounds or more of weight plates inside your vehicle. You will have an almost impossible time keeping the plates from slipping and sliding around in your vehicle. And if you are moving at speed and have to stomp on the breaks ... well ... where do I send the flowers?

Olympic weight plate tree:

If the weight plate tree you choose is disassembled, boxed, and will fit into your vehicle, I recommend picking it up yourself. This is provided you can find it locally for less than or equal to the lowest online price. Do not forget to factor in the online shipping costs.

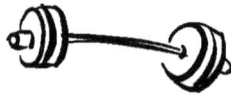

4. Outfitting Up your Gym

5

SETTING UP YOUR GYM

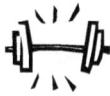

Getting the equipment into your gym

Make sure you know the dimensions of the door opening your equipment will have to pass through in order to be placed inside your gym. If you live in an apartment building or if your gym is on any floor other than ground level, do not forget to take into account the negotiation of stairs and/or small elevators. Regardless of where you live, when fully assembled, the larger pieces of equipment are heavy and cumbersome. You do not want to injure yourself trying to shift them.

Treadmill:
It is best to let trained personnel place your treadmill where you want it. They do it for a living and will know where best to hold the treadmill for a balanced carry.

Power Rack:
The Power Rack when assembled weighs over 300 pounds, so carry it piece by piece into your gym area and put it together there.

Olympic weight plate tree:
The Olympic weight plate tree will be delivered flat in a box. It is an awkward piece to handle when fully assembled, so be sure to do the assembly in your gym space.

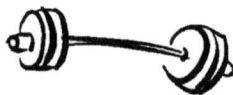

Tools for setting up your equipment

Note: The following tools are used in the assembly of the makes and models of equipment discussed in this book. Equipment not discussed in this book may require different tools for assembly.

Treadmill:
If you decide to forgo delivery and want to set the treadmill up yourself, here are the tools you will need.

- One 5/32-inch hex key wrench (also known as an Allen wrench, one came with the treadmill).
- One 9/16-inch combination wrench. (A combination wrench has two ends. One end of this wrench looks like the letter U, the other end like the letter O. Either end can be used to tighten or loosen bolts. Make sure both ends are noted as 9/16. This wrench does not come with the treadmill.)
- One Phillips head screwdriver.

Power Rack:
Clear instructions are included with the rack, and it is relatively easy to setup. I say relatively easy because one person can do it alone, but it is much easier with another set of hands.

Tools you will need are:

- One ¾-inch socket.
- One ⅞-inch socket.
- One socket wrench (also known as a ratchet wrench).
- One 15/16-inch capacity crescent wrench (also known as an adjustable wrench).

If after assembling the rack you find it is not level (rocks front to back at opposite corners) place a couple of wooden shims under one of the corners.

The concrete floor in my basement is not perfectly level so I have placed shims under my Power Rack. I use over 800 pounds within my rack and the shims hold up with no problems.

Alternatively, you can spend most of your day or week trying to level your Power Rack. You can also bolt it to the floor like most commercial gyms do. Try the shims first. The shims are available at home improvement stores. You may want to paint the shims black to help them blend-in.

Olympic weight plate tree:
Tools needed:

- One ¾-inch socket.
- One ⅞-inch socket.

- One socket wrench (also known as a ratchet wrench).
- One 15/16-inch capacity crescent wrench (also known as an adjustable wrench).

*Be sure to check your equipment's warrantee information sheet, it will tell you exactly what is covered and for how many years. You may even find you are entitled to free in-home service. Keep all of your equipment warrantees in a safe place, and filed where you can easily find them if they are needed.

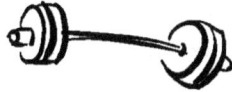

Upkeep and maintenance procedures

As the proud owner of a home gym, you are responsible for its upkeep and cleanliness. They may be unsavory duties, but they are necessary.

Dumbbell handles:

A ⅜-inch Allen wrench (also known as a hex key wrench) will be needed to periodically tighten the ends of the dumbbell handles. This wrench must be purchased separately. I bought mine from a home improvement store. Keep the Allen wrench in your gym so it is always handy.

Power Rack:

- Every six months, tighten all of the bolts and nuts that hold the Power Rack together. They may not need tightening, but check them anyway.
- Check the Rack for chipped paint and touch-up those areas using an artist's brush and a small amount of paint. Rustoleum is a good brand.

A 7-foot Olympic-style weightlifting bar:

- Tighten the ends if necessary.
- Replace torn weightlifting bar/safety rod protector wraps with a new set.

Floor:

- Clean floors as needed. It is easier and better to clean as you go than to wait until the end of the week.
- A vacuum works great for cleaning up chalk dust.
- A damp sponge-mop or rag removes perspiration.
- Remember to clean the space under the treadmill.

Gym walls and ceiling:

Lint, dust, and spider silk accumulates on all of the surfaces within the gym and should be removed. Once a week, wipe down or vacuum the walls and ceiling. Yeah, I know this sounds like overkill, but it will only take a few minutes to do. It will greatly improve your gym's air quality.

Air Filter:

- If you have chosen to get a room air filter, and I hope you have, regularly change the filter per the manufacturer's instructions. Do not try vacuuming the filter and putting it back into the filter housing, vacuuming does not work on most micron filters.
- Clean the filter housing.
- Keep a couple of clean filters on hand if you can. The store is bound to be out of stock when you need a quick replacement. You may find an inexpensive source for filters on the Internet.

Lighting:

Make sure you have a couple of replacement bulbs or tubes handy.

Treadmill:

- Wipe down the treadmill after each use. To decrease the possibility of getting moisture where you do not want it, spray the cleanser onto a cleaning rag and not directly onto the treadmill.
- Check the tension of your treadmill's striding belt when you are wiping down the treadmill. If the belt is loose or has slewed left or right, tighten it. Your user's manual will show you how to tighten the belt, and an Allen wrench should have come with your treadmill for this purpose.

- If you have problems with your treadmill, such as a part needing replacement, check the warrantee information to see if the part is still under warrantee. It is important to address problems as soon as you notice them.

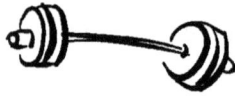

5. SETTING UP YOUR GYM

SMALL GYM BIG WORKOUTS

6

SAFETY MEASURES

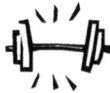

Safety Measures

I am a lone-lifter, and in the over 30 years that I have been working out, I have been injury free. "How is this possible?" you ask.

I:

- Wear the appropriate attire for gym sessions.
- Wear my weightlifting belt when lifting.
- Always respect the equipment, realizing the injuries that could result if improperly handled.
- Make sure my shoes are properly tied. I've seen many people trip and get injured in the gym because of an untied shoelace.
- Use weightlifting chalk to maintain a firm grip on the equipment.
- Maintain strict form when lifting weights, walking, and running.
- Never workout when I'm too tired to concentrate properly.
- Buy and use only sturdy equipment.
- Never leave a piece of equipment where it may become a tripping hazard.
- Always use collars on the weight bars, so the weight plates do not slide off.
- Quickly inspect any equipment before I use it.
- Always use the Power Rack's safety rods.
- Never go for my one-rep-max.
- Warm up slowly.
- Generally do not push beyond the specification of a

given piece of equipment, barbells have been the exception.

- Keep a towel handy to wipe off perspiration that drips onto equipment, lest it become a slipping hazard.
- Do not talk on the phone while I'm working-out.

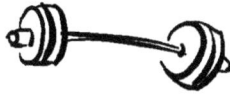

7

COMMERCIAL AND MILITARY GYM ETIQUETTE

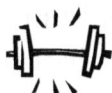

Small Gym Big Workouts has detailed everything you need to know to set up and maintain a gym in your home. However, there may be times when, for whatever reason, you will want to workout at a gym other than your own. If this is so, there are some simple rules of etiquette to remember:

- Always be respectful of the gym's equipment, facilities, and patrons.
- Once you have finished using equipment, return it to its proper place.
- Wipe down the equipment you have used when you are finished with it.
- Grunting is sometimes unavoidable when lifting weights, but try to avoid unnecessary yelling and using foul language as it may disrupt the workouts of others.
- Do not bang the weights.
- Do not modify cable machines by adding dumbbells to the weight stack.
- Between sets, do not leave dumbbells and barbells where people may trip over them.
- Always lay a clean towel over weight benches before using them, and wipe them down with available cleaner after use.
- Never chat with a person when they are actively working their muscles. It breaks their concentration and injuries could result. If the person is between sets, just wave to them. They will come over to you, or beckon you over if they wish to converse. In any case, try to keep chatting to a minimum, as you both should be

there to workout. If there is a lot to say, arrange to meet away from the gym.

- Do not lounge on equipment if you have no plans to use it. Others are waiting for it.
- If you use weight lifting chalk, cleanup after yourself. If you make a mess and leave it, the gym may outlaw the use of chalk altogether.
- Please, please cover your mouth with your towel or tissue when you cough or sneeze.
- Please, please, please do not use the towel you have just sneezed in to wipe off the equipment you have just finished using. Yes, I have seen this. If you know you are ill, keep tissue handy and dispose of it properly after use.
- Try really hard not to use your cell phone.
- Wear only clean-soled shoes in the gym.
- Avoid injury to yourself or others. Remember to observe gym safety and leave the gym on your own two feet, not on a stretcher.

These are all just basic courtesies and I am sure they are second nature to you. So wherever you decide to workout, work hard, work consistently, and have fun.

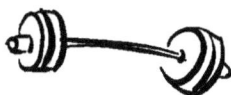

SMALL GYM BIG WORKOUTS

8

EXERCISE EXAMPLES

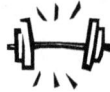

Many different exercises can be performed with the gym set-up described in this book. Every muscle group can be worked. A short listing is included here to get you started.

If you are not familiar with how to perform an exercise listed here, search the Internet using the exercise name to find proper technique descriptions.

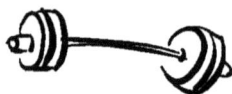

Exercise list

Neck:
- Weighted Neck Extensions (forward, back, left, and right sides using the Headstrap Made for Hercules)
- Exercise Band Neck Extensions (in conjunction with the Headstrap Made for Hercules)

Traps:
- Barbell Shrugs (holding the bar in front of you)
- Barbell Shrugs (holding the bar behind you while in the power rack and using the safety rods)
- Dumbbell Shrugs (while standing or seated)
- Upright Barbell Rows
- Upright Dumbbell Rows
- Straight-Armed Dips

Shoulders:
- Standing Military Press (aka Barbell Press)
- Seated Military Press

- Plate Raises
- Lateral Dumbbell Raises
- Front Dumbbell Raises
- Bent-Over Laterals (Dumbbells)
- Inverted Flyes (Dumbbells)
- Seated Dumbbell Press (one arm at a time or both together)
- Standing Dumbbell Press (one arm at a time or both together)
- Arnold Dumbbell Press
- Front Barbell Raises
- Upright Barbell Rows
- Upright Olympic Curl Bar Rows
- Upright Dumbbell Rows
- Bent-Over Barbell Rows
- Bent-Over Dumbbell Rows
- Dips (bodyweight)
- Dips (weighted)
- Rotator Cuff Exercises using Exercise Bands
- Rotator Cuff Exercises using Weight Plates
- Rotator Cuff Exercises using Dumbbell

Triceps:
- Close-Grip Bench Press
- Lying Barbell Triceps Extensions
- Lying Dumbbell Triceps Extensions
- Skull Crushers using the Olympic Curl Bar
- Dumbbell Kickbacks
- Barbell French Curls

- Dumbbell French Curls (one arm at a time or both together)
- Dips (bodyweight and using dip bar handles in power rack)
- Dips (weighted and using dip bar handles in power rack)
- Bench Dips
- Pushups (using pushup handles)

Biceps:
- Barbell Standing Curls
- Close Grip Curls
- Wide Grip Curls
- Barbell Seated Curls
- Olympic Curl Bar Curls
- Alternate Dumbbell Curls (standing)
- Alternate Dumbbell Curls (seated)
- Dumbbell Curls (both arms at the same time)
- Seated Incline Dumbbell Curls
- Spider Curls
- Reverse Barbell Curls
- Reverse Olympic Curl Bar Curls
- Reverse Dumbbell Curls
- Reverse Incline Bench Curls
- Hammer Curls (both arms at the same time)
- Hammer Curls (alternating arms)
- Across-the-Body Hammer Curls (alternating arms)
- Preacher Curls
- One-Arm Preacher Curls
- Scott Curls

- Drag Curls
- Concentration Curls

Elbows:
- Elbow Warm-ups using Resistance Bands
- Elbow Warm-ups using 2.5-, 5-, and 10-Pound Weight Plates

Forearms:
- Barbell Forearm Curls (Stand with barbell in front of you aka Wrist Curls.)
- Standing behind the Back Wrist Curl (using power rack and safety rods)
- Seated Barbell Wrist Curls
- Seated Reverse Barbell Wrist Curls
- Dumbbell Wrist Curls
- Wrist Curls using Olympic Curl Bar
- Reverse Curls using Olympic Curl Bar

Hands:
- Grip Strengthener (Grab onto chin-up bar and hold your weight until your grip fails.)

Chest:
- Flat Barbell Bench Press
- Wide Grip Bench Press
- Incline Barbell Bench Press
- Decline Barbell Bench Press
- Flat Dumbbell Bench Press
- Incline Dumbbell Bench Press

- Decline Dumbbell Bench Press
- Flat Dumbbell Flyes
- Incline Dumbbell Flyes
- Decline Dumbbell Flyes
- Dips (bodyweight)
- Dips (weighted)
- Bent-Arm Pullovers (Barbell or Olympic Curl Bar)
- Straight-Arm Pullovers (Barbell or Olympic Curl Bar)
- Pushups (using pushup handles)

Back:
- Deadlifts
- Half Deadlifts
- Romanian Deadlifts
- Stiff-Leg Deadlifts
- One Handed Deadlifts (using cable handle, carabiner and loading pin)
- Bent Over Barbell Rows
- Bent Over Dumbbell Rows
- Bent Over One Arm Barbell Rows
- Bent Over One Arm Dumbbell Rows
- Reverse Incline Dumbbell Rows
- Barbell Shrugs
- Dumbbell Shrugs
- Chin-ups (wide, medium, and close grips)
- Pull-ups (wide, medium, and close grips)
- Barbell High Pulls
- Dumbbell High Pulls
- Upright Rows
- Bent Over Dumbbell Flyes

- Reverse Incline Dumbbell Flyes
- Reverse Incline Barbell Rows
- Reverse Incline Barbell Shrugs
- Reverse Incline Dumbbell Rows
- Reverse Incline Dumbbell Shrugs
- Power Cleans
- Back Extensions on Exercise Ball
- Good Mornings

Abdominals:
- Sit-ups
- Exercise Ball Sit-ups
- Reverse Sit-ups (aka Leg Lifts)
- Sit-ups hanging over the edge of a bench (You'll have to anchor your feet for this one.)
- Decline Sit-ups
- Knee Raises
- Hanging Leg Raises
- Exercise Ball Crunches
- Weighted Abdominal Crunches
- Incline Reverse Crunches

Legs:
- Olympic Squats (wide, intermediate, and narrow stances)
- Powerlifting Squats
- Box Squats
- Front Squats
- Jefferson Squat (using barbell)
- Half Squats

- Dumbbell Squats
- Sissy Squats
- Barbell Hack Squats
- Barbell Deadlifts
- Dumbbell Deadlifts
- Stiff-Leg Deadlifts
- Barbell Lunge Squat
- Dumbbell Lunge Squat
- Lunge Walking (using either a barbell or dumbbells)
- Farmers Walk
- Leg Extensions
- Hamstring Curls (aka leg curls)
- Calf Raises
- Standing Barbell behind the back Calf Raises
- Donkey Raises (using dip belt, carabiner and loading pin)
- Seated Calf Raises
- Adductor Exercises using Exercise Bands
- Abductor Exercises using Exercise Bands
- Gluteus maximus Exercises using Exercise Bands
- Tibialis Exercises
- Jumping Rope

Ankles:
- Jumping Rope
- Calf Raises (standing or seated and using weight)
- Ankle Curls (holding dumbbell between feet)
- Ankle Extensions With Exercise Bands (up, down, left, and right sides)

Feet:

- Barefoot Calf Raises (holding a dumbbell in one or both hands)
- Barefoot Walking on Toes (with light dumbbell in each hand)
- Barefoot Walking on Heels (with light dumbbell in each hand)
- Barefoot Forefoot Press (Using exercise ball, place ball against a wall or solid object, with heels on floor, forefoot against the ball, and legs straight, press forefoot and toes into the ball slowly ten times for three sets. Do these while seated on the floor or on a chair.)

Resistance Bands:

- Neck Extensions (in combination with Headstrap Made for Hercules)
- Resisted Pushup
- Chest Press
- Overhead Flyes
- Upright Rows
- Rear Delt Pull
- Deadlifts
- Half Deadlifts
- Back Extensions
- Bent Over Rows
- Seated Rows
- Shoulder Shrugs
- Front Raise
- Lateral Raise
- Biceps Curl

- Reverse Curls
- Forearm Curls
- Triceps Kickbacks
- Abdominal Twists
- Resistance Crunchers
- Squats
- Lunge
- Single-Leg Kickbacks
- Hamstring Curls
- Single-Side Leg Press
- Leg Extensions
- Seated Calf Raises
- Adductors (Inner Thighs)
- Abductors (Outer Thighs)
- Standing Side Bend
- Rotator Cuff Warm-up and Strengthening

Exercise Ball:
- Pushups
- Prone Ball Roll
- Sit-ups
- Lateral Obliques
- Back Extensions
- Reverse Back Extensions
- Hip Extensions
- Lower Back Roll
- Inner Thigh Squeeze
- Wall Squat
- Hamstring Curls
- Lower Back Lift

- Abdominal Curls
- Arm and Leg Lifts
- Bounce Up And Down
- Side-to-Side Hip
- Clockwise Circles
- Counter-Clockwise Circles
- Back Bridge
- Back Bridge With One Leg Raised
- Front Bridge
- Front Bridge With Walkout
- Lunge Back
- Pike
- Tuck
- Ball Pass

Aerobics:
- Interval Work on the Treadmill
- Speed Bag Work
- Jump Rope
- Punching Bag Work
- Aerobic DVDs and tapes played in your DVD/VCR player
- Cross Fit Circuit Training
- Calisthenics

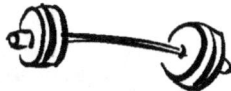

Mack shows you Major Muscle Group Workouts

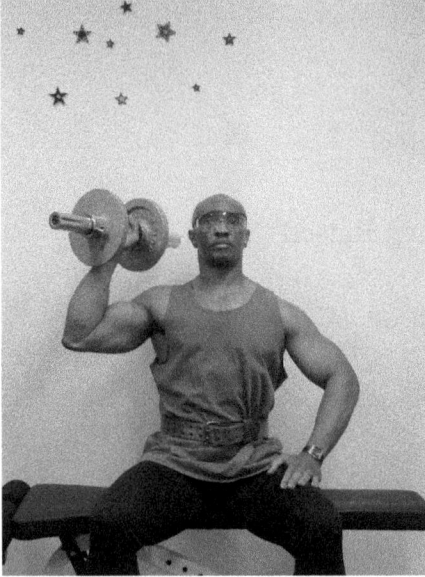

Seated One-Arm Dumbbell Shoulder Press

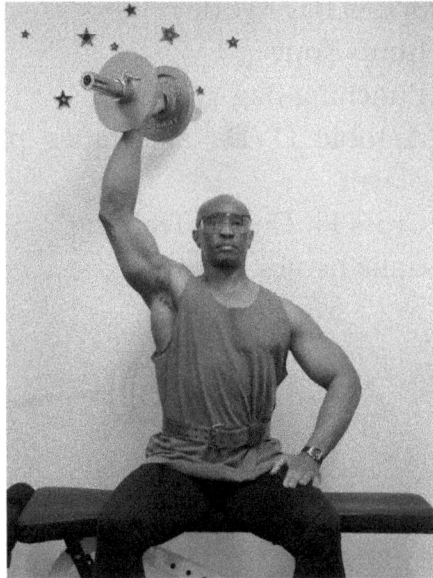

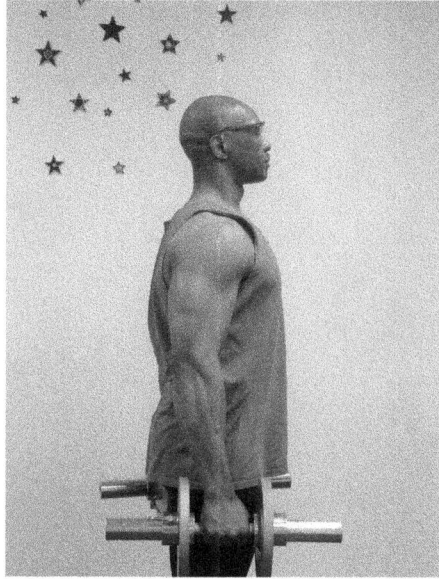

Standing Rear
Deltoids with
Dumbbells

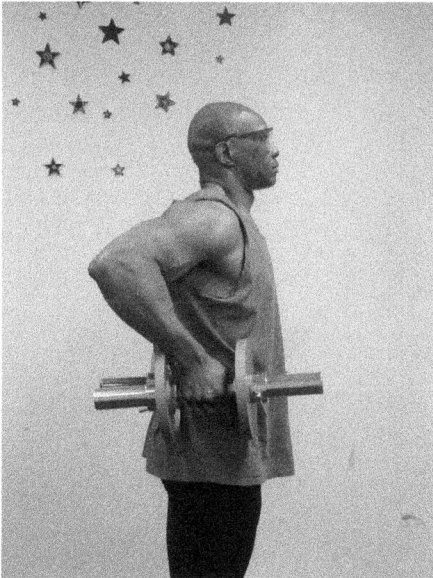

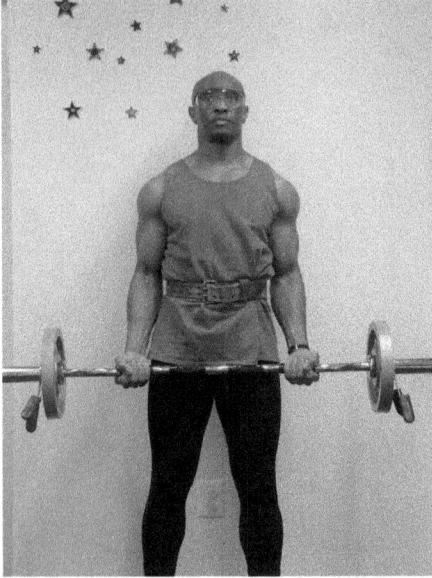

Biceps Curl with
Olympic Curl
Bar

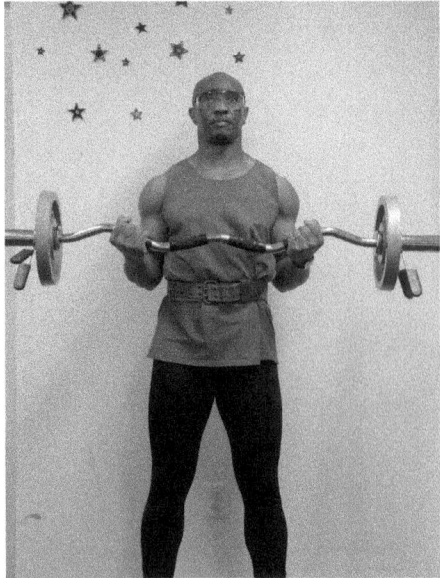

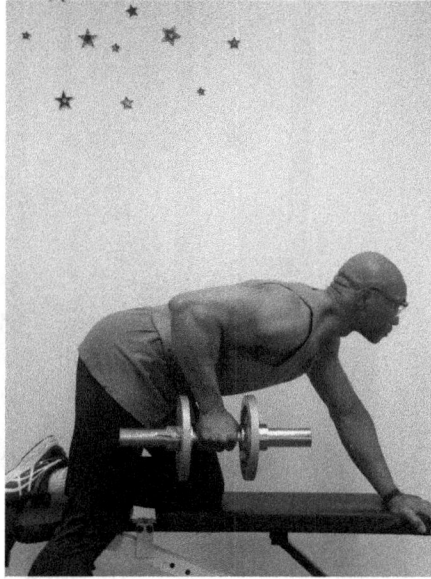

Triceps
Dumbbell
Kickbacks

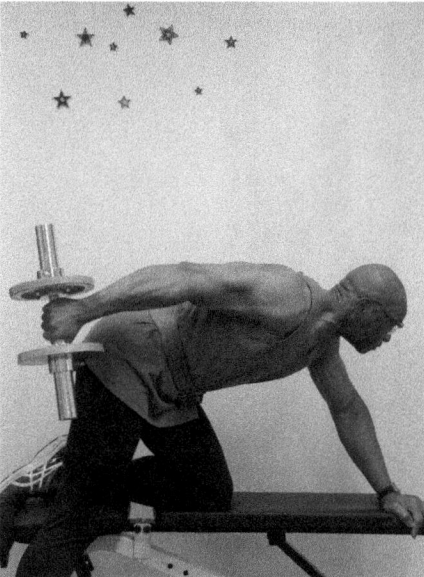

119

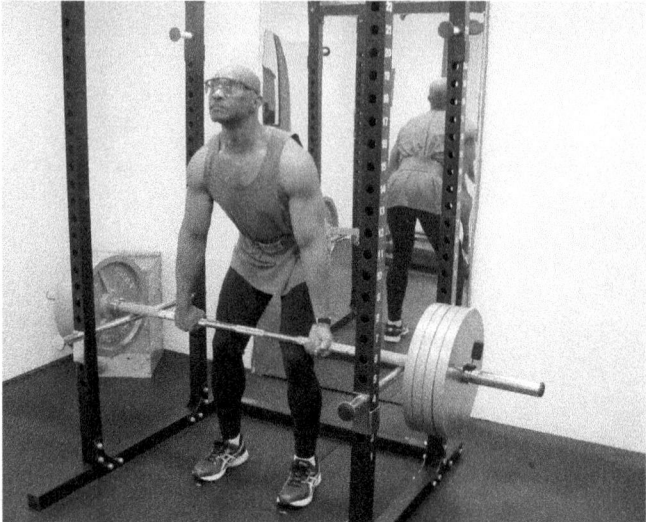

Half Deadlifts
for back in
Power Rack

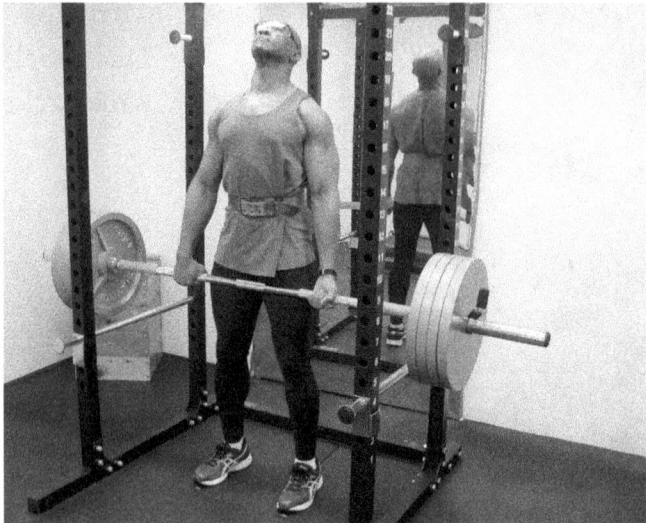

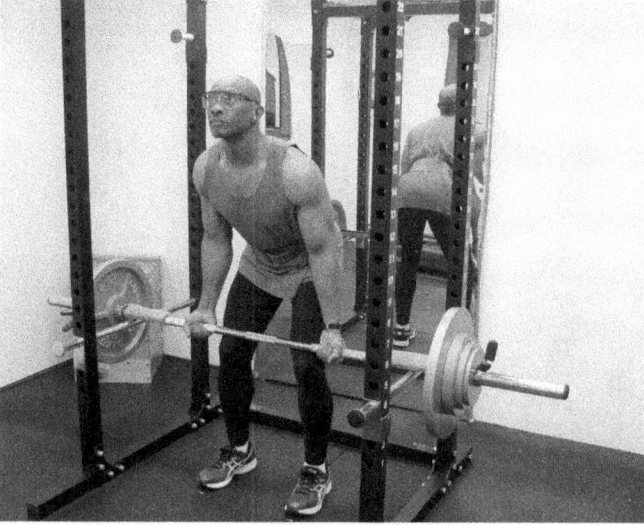

Bent over
Barbell Rows
for back

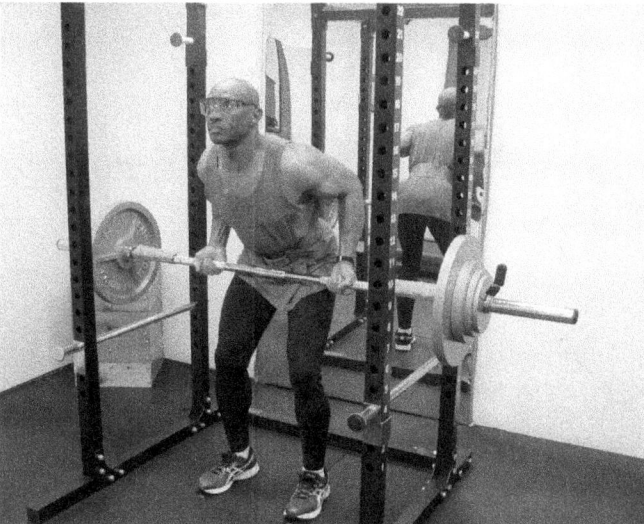

121

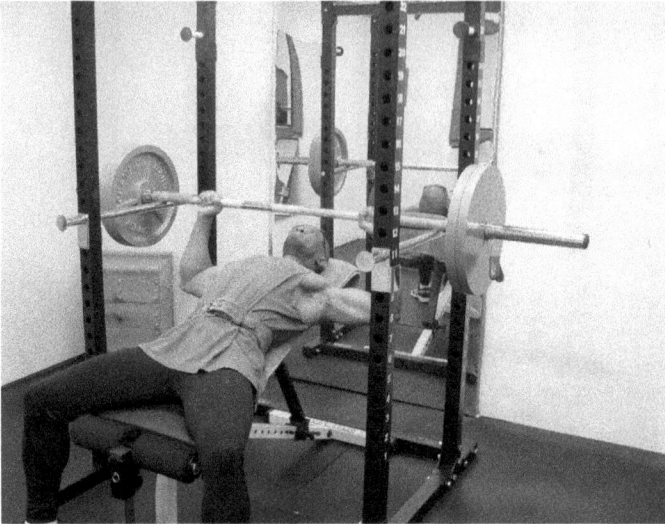

Incline Barbell
Bench Press for
chest

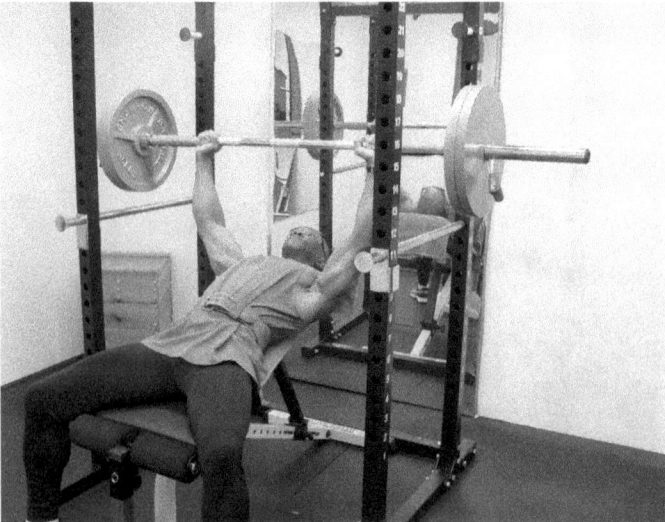

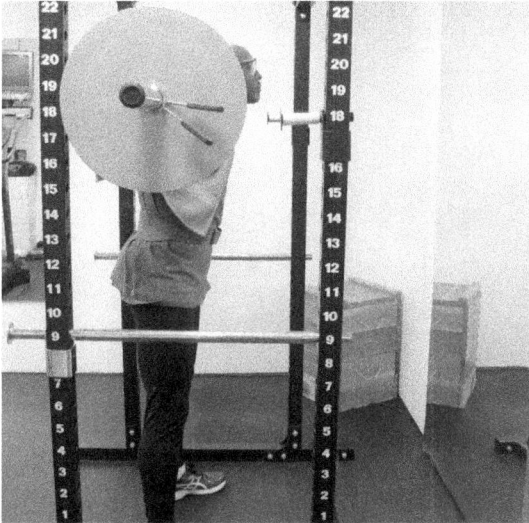

Powerlifting
Squats
for legs

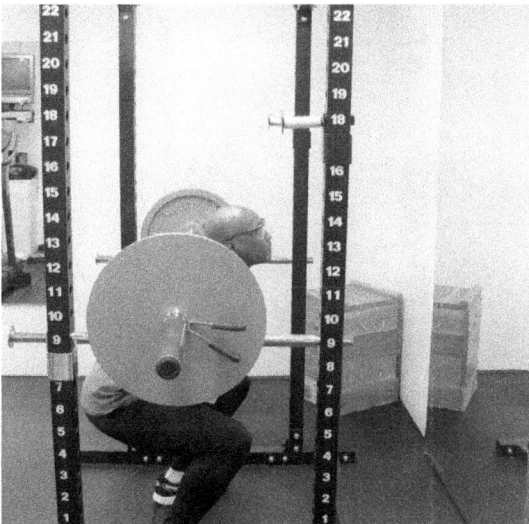

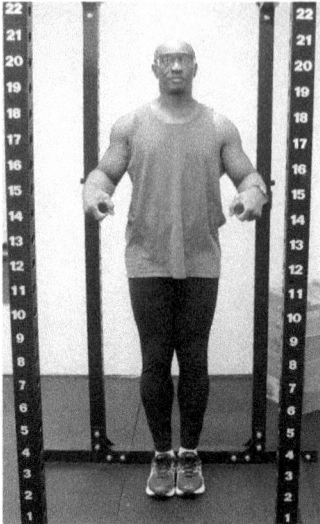

Hanging Leg
Raises for abs
using dip bar
handles

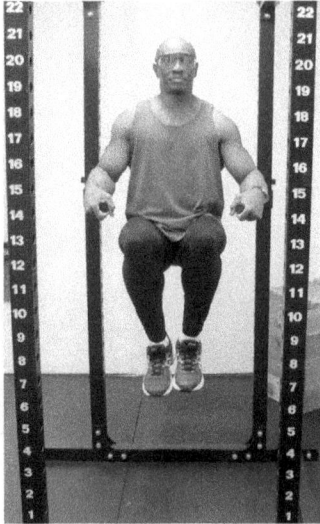

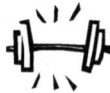

8. EXERCISES EXAMPLES

Meet the Author

Mack Webb has been lifting weights since high school. He is a physical fitness enthusiast who knows improving physical fitness can also help improve quality of life. Mack is an Army veteran and a world traveler who enjoys learning new things. His affinity for the outdoors prompted him to pursue and complete a degree in Horticulture at the University of Maryland. Mack and his wife, Celia, have authored ten books and even now are more than likely hammering away at their keyboards in Virginia's peaceful horse country. When not writing, publishing, or working out in their own home gym, they pull on their Wellingtons and busy themselves in their large organic garden.

www.ingramcontent.com/pod-product-compliance
Lightning Source LLC
Chambersburg PA
CBHW060806050426
42449CB00008B/1557